The Conduction System of the Mammalian Heart

An Anatomico-histological Study of the Atrioventricular Bundle and the Purkinje Fibers

CARDIOPULMONARY MEDICINE FROM IMPERIAL COLLEGE PRESS

Series Editor: Robert H. Anderson
National Heart & Lung Institute, London

Published:

Controversies in the Description of Congenitally Malformed Hearts
(*with video*)
    R. H. Anderson

The Conduction System in the Mammalian Heart — An Anatomico-
histological Study of the Atrioventricular Bundle and the Purkinje Fibers
    S. Tawara; translated by K. Suma & M. Shimada

Forthcoming:

Echocardiography in Congenital Heart Disease Made Simple
    S. Y. Ho, A. N. Redington, M. L. Rigby & R. H. Anderson

Fetal Electrocardiography
    E. M. Symonds, D. Sahota & A. Chang

Cardiopulmonary Medicine from Imperial College Press

The Conduction System of the Mammalian Heart

An Anatomico-histological Study of the Atrioventricular Bundle and the Purkinje Fibers

S. Tawara
foreword by L. Aschoff

Translated by

Kozo Suma
Munehiro Shimada
preface by R. H. Anderson

Imperial College Press

Published by

Imperial College Press
57 Shelton Street
Covent Garden
London WC2H 9HE

Distributed by

World Scientific Publishing Co. Pte. Ltd.
5 Toh Tuck Link, Singapore 596224
USA office: 27 Warren Street, Suite 401-402, Hackensack, NJ 07601
UK office: 57 Shelton Street, Covent Garden, London WC2H 9HE

British Library Cataloguing-in-Publication Data
A catalogue record for this book is available from the British Library.

ISBN-13 978-1-86094-116-0
ISBN-10 1-86094-116-8

DAS REIZLEITUNGSSYSTEM
DES SÄUGETIERHERZENS.

EINE ANATOMISCH-HISTOLOGISCHE STUDIE
ÜBER DAS ATRIOVENTRIKULARBÜNDEL
UND DIE PURKINJESCHEN FÄDEN.

VON

DR. S. TAWARA

JAPAN.

MIT EINEM VORWORT

VON **L. ASCHOFF** (MARBURG).

MIT 5 LITHOGRAPHISCHEN UND 5 LICHTDRUCK-TAFELN
SOWIE 2 ABBILDUNGEN IM TEXT.

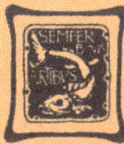

VERLAG VON GUSTAV FISCHER IN JENA.
1906.

Facsimile cover of S. Tawara's original monograph in German

Contents

Preface

The conduction system of the heart is very much a twentieth century structure. Parts of the system had certainly been seen in the nineteenth century and, with present day knowledge, it is easy to recognize drawings from this period showing the atrioventricular bundle on the crest of the ventricular septum. The so-called Purkinje cells had also been recognized within the ventricular subendocardium, and had been the source of numerous discussions concerning their potential function. By the end of the century, accounts had appeared describing an atrioventricular bundle[1] but, in the self-same year as His's study, another investigator claimed to have demonstrated multiple pathways of conduction for the normal cardiac impulse across the right atrioventricular groove.[2] This, then, was the state of knowledge when Sunao Tawara arrived in Marburg to study with Ludwig Aschoff, already recognized as an expert in anatomic pathology and soon, with Mönckeberg, to become a giant in this field of study.

The fruits of Tawara's labors are considerable. Together with Aschoff, he discovered the nodule which is now recognized as being diagnostic for rheumatic involvement of the heart, and which now bears Aschoff's name. Aschoff, however, was particularly interested in establishing the substrate for the muscular decompensation known to occur in the failing heart. He had the notion that this may involve the recently discovered muscular bundle connecting the atrial and ventricular muscle masses. As it turns out, the results of the investigations carried out by Tawara on this topic had consequences far beyond the realms of cardiac failure. In reality, as the reader of this book will see, the anatomic studies of Tawara laid the basis for the development of the science of cardiac electrophysiology.

The detailed studies of electrical activation of the heart, although triggered by the pioneering studies of those such as Einthoven, Lewis, Meek and Wilson, did not reach fruition until the last quarter of this century. And, even now, controversies continue with regard to the precise anatomic substrates for atrioventricular conduction and its abnormalities, with some present day accounts[3,4] differing markedly from the initial studies of Tawara. How can this be?

The explanation is simple. Tawara published an initial account of his studies in markedly abbreviated form,[5] this reference representing little more than an abstract of a paper presented at a learned symposium. He chose to describe the body of his researches in a monograph published in 1906 by the house of Gustav Fischer in Jena. At first sight, the monograph is daunting. It is made up of 200 pages of densely written scientific German, punctuated only here and there by rudimentary diagrams. This was my first impression of the book when, in 1963, as a medical student, I examined the copy in the Manchester Medical Library while preparing a thesis for an intercalated year of anatomy during my medical studies. I failed to discover the beautifully tinted plates which were hidden under the back cover of the slender volume. These first became apparent to me in 1974 when, with Anton Becker and Geil Janse, we began to conduct anatomic–electrophysiologic correlations in animal and human hearts.[6,7] Even then, however, we delved merely cursorily into the dense German text, translating only those passages which seemed pertinent to our own accounts of the atrioventricular junctional area of the human heart. These brief incursions, however, made us well aware that our own findings served very much as an endorsement of Tawara's studies, but we were unaware of the true extent of Tawara's knowledge. What we would have given for the full translation which you, the reader, now hold in your hands. And, had this translation been available five, or thirty-five, years ago, would we have avoided our recent controversies[3,4]? Who can tell? What we certainly can now do is appreciate the breadth of the studies conducted by Tawara, and the accuracy of his observations. As Keith stated in his autobiography,[8] with the discovery of the conducting system of Tawara, heart research entered a new epoch. We can now enjoy the writings which ushered in this epoch.

For this, we owe a huge debt to Kozo Suma and Munehiro Shimada, who have diligently translated the original German first into Japanese, and now into English. I have tried to make my own contribution to this venture by editing the English translation. I have tried to stick as closely as possible to the direct translation, but also to give the text some style and "flow." The end result, to me, reads remarkably well, but I am obviously biased! At all events, we can now all share the amazing results of Tawara's efforts, which truly are epochal.

Robert H. Anderson
London, April 1999

References

1. His, W., Jr. Die Tätigkeit des embryonalen Herzens und deren Bedeutung für die Lehre von der Herzbewegung beim Erwachsenen *Arb aus d med Klinik zu Leipzig* (1893), pp. 14–60.
2. Kent, A.F.S. Researches on the structure and function of the mammalian heart, *J. Physiol.*, 1983;14:233–254.
3. James, T.N. Morphology of the human atrioventricular node, with remarks pertinent to its electrophysiology, *Am. Heart J.*, 1961;62:756–771.
4. Racker, D.K. Atrioventricular node and input pathways: a correlated gross anatomical and histological study of the canine atrioventricular junctional region, *Anat. Rec.*, 1989;224:336–354.
5. Tawara, S. Über die sogenannten abnormen Sehnenfäden des Herzens; ein Beitrag zur Pathologie des Reizleitungssystems des Herzens (*Beitr z path Anat u z allg Path*, Jena, 1906).
6. Anderson, R.H., Janse, M.J., van Capelle, F.J.L., Billette J., Becker A.E., Durrer D. A combined morphologic and electrophysiologic study of the atrioventricular node of the rabbit heart, *Circ. Res.*, 1974;35: 909–920.
7. Janse, M.J., Anderson, R.H., van Capelle, F.J.L., Durrer, D. A combined electrophysiological and anatomical study of the human fetal heart, *Am. Heart J.*, 1976;91:556–562.
8. Keith, A. *An Autobiography* (Watts & Co., London, 1950), pp. 254–259.

Translators' Note

Sunao Tawara's epoch-making work[6-9] on the excitation conduction system of the mammalian heart was done at Ludwig Aschoff's Pathological Institute in Marburg, Germany. It paved the way for the advancement of modern cardiology. Together with the development of electrocardiography, which took place about the same time, the elucidation of this system made a significant contribution to cardiology.

Tawara's careful and precise account of the conduction system from the atrioventricular node through the His–Purkinje system to the ordinary ventricular muscle fibers was based on both light microscopic and macroscopic observation; its anatomical significance and physiological inferences were rapidly acknowledged by the specialists in the field — it retains, even today, all of its original actuality. Research on the conduction system constitutes a major field for future study in cardiology, particularly in the area of arrhythmology, and the pioneering work done by Tawara will surely serve as a reference for both basic and clinical research in the years ahead.

In 1987, the German original of Tawara's monograph[6] was reprinted in Japan by the Committee for Reprinting Tawara's Monograph with the permission of Gustav Fischer Verlag, Stuttgart. In 1990, a Japanese translation was published by Maruzen Co., Ltd. The present English translation was prepared in the hope of assisting cardiological researchers around the world; its publication is a matter of great joy for the translators.

Tawara was born in Oita Prefecture on the island of Kyushu in 1873. After graduating from the Faculty of Medicine, the University of Tokyo, in 1901, he went to Germany in 1903 for further studies at his father's expense and spent the next three years researching myocarditis[1,2] and the conduction system[6–9] at Aschoff's laboratory. Tawara's work on myocarditis is also referred to in Aschoff's foreword and in the introduction to the monograph by Tawara himself. It is to be mentioned that the Aschoff body[1,2] in rheumatic myocarditis was discovered during Tawara's study, directed by Aschoff, on myocarditis. The references of this translators' note contain the treatises of Tawara on the conduction system of the heart,[6–9] Aschoff's article *"Zur Myocarditisfrage,"*[1] Aschoff and Tawara's book on myocarditis,[2] and some other material concerning Aschoff and Tawara. Tawara returned to Japan in 1906 and served as Professor of Pathology at Kyushu University from 1908 until his retirement in 1933. During that period, he also served as President of the Japan Pathological Association for two terms. In 1952, he died at the age of 78.

Recently, the texts of six letters written by Tawara to Aschoff[4] were released, and they evoked a great response. Besides affording a glimpse at the warm master–student relationship, these missives provide a vivid picture of the dedication and hardships of a Japanese scholar, studying abroad at the beginning of the 20th century and attempting to make scientific achievements.

In his letter dated October 8, 1905, to Aschoff, Tawara wrote: "…when I on a quiet evening sat in my digs and thought of my father, who, I am sure, every day and every hour thought of me in quiet hope of my success, and when I then considered the failure of my experiments, I was deeply unhappy. During these two long years I did not have one single happy day. After we had this spring made a new discovery on the connecting bundle, I regained a little hope,…" Prof. Dr. Jürgen Aschoff,[4] L. Aschoff's son, mentioned that there seemed to have been, despite many differences in temperament, a congeniality in character and view of life, particularly in feelings of gratitude for, and of duty towards, their fathers between the professor and his student. This is reflected in Aschoff's letter[3] dated April 16, 1906, just at the time of publication of the monograph, to his father. It reads: "For an Easter gift this year, I will send you a book recently written by Dr. Tawara, who conducted investigations of the heart at my laboratory for two-and-one-half years. Indeed, this book is the result of the tremendous industriousness on the part of this Japanese scholar. I present it to you as my sincere thanks for your support and encouragement, which allowed me to further my professional career..."

In recalling Tawara, his teacher, Tamaki Imai[5] (Professor of Pathology, Kyushu University), wrote: "...There are some who often talk very proudly about their academic achievements. However, this kind of presumptuousness was foreign to Tawara. He very seldom spoke about his achievements, and then only at the strong request of his students."

It is noteworthy that this year the Aschoff–Tawara exhibition has been inaugurated at the Institute for Anatomy and Cell Biology, which is housed in the building of the former Aschoff's Pathological Institute of the Philipps-University of Marburg, and that a symposium has been held on this occasion. These have been realized through the efforts of Prof. Horst F. Kern and Prof. Gerhard Aumüller.

The publication of this English translation would not have been possible without the help of a great many parties. We are particularly grateful to Prof. Robert H. Anderson, who wrote the preface to this translation, proofread the manuscript, and was of invaluable assistance in the publication. We are indebted to Prof. Tatsuo Shimada, who participated in reprinting the German original and publishing the Japanese translation, as well as to Drs. Wolfgang R. Ade and Andrew J. Parry, who supported the publication of the English translation in many ways. We are also very grateful to Prof. Motokazu Hori for his warm encouragement for this project. The photograph of Tawara was kindly provided by Dr. Satoru Murayama, Tawara's grandson, and that of Aschoff by the Pathological Institute of the Philipps-University of Marburg. Thanks are also due to Mrs. Noriko Sunohara for her skillful secretarial support. Last but not least, we would like to express our deep gratitude to Gustav Fischer Verlag for their permission to publish this English translation.

Kozo Suma, M.D.
Munehiro Shimada, M.D.

Tokyo, September 1999

References

1. Aschoff, L. Zur Myocarditisfrage. *Verhandl d deutsch path Gesellsch* 1904;8:46–53.
2. Aschoff, L., und Tawara, S. *Die heutige Lehre von den pathologisch-anatomischen Grundlagen der Herzschwäche* (Verlag von Gustav Fischer, Jena, 1906).
3. *Ludwig Aschoff–Ein Gelehrtenleben in Briefen an die Familie* (Hans Fernand Schulz Verlag, Freiburg im Breisgau, 1966), pp. 175–176.
4. Aschoff, J. Sunao Tawara, one of Ludwig Aschoff's most prominent Japanese scholars. In *Selection from Tawara's Monograph: The Conduction System of the Mammalian Heart*, eds. Suma K., Shimada, M., Shimada, T., *et al.*, Organizing Committee of V Asia–Pacific Symposium on Cardiac Pacing and Electrophysiology and VIII Annual Meeting of the Japanese Society of Cardiac Pacing and Electrophysiology, Tokyo, 1993, pp. 45–61.
5. Imai, T. Scientific achievements of Tawara, *Kyudai Iho* 1952;22(2): 2–4.
6. Tawara, S. *Das Reizleitungssystem des Säugetierherzens. Eine anatomisch–histologische Studie über das Atrioventrikularbündel und die Purkinjeschen Fäden* (Verlag von Gustav Fischer, Jena, 1906).
7. Tawara, S. Die Topographie und Histologie der Brückenfasern. Ein Beitrag zur Lehre von der Bedeutung der Purkinjeschen Fäden. *Zentralbl f Physiol* 1905;19:70–76.
8. Tawara, S. Anatomisch-histologische Nachprüfung der Schnittführung an den von Prof. H.E. Hering übersandten Hundeherzen. *Arch f d ges Physiol* 1906;111:300–302.
9. Tawara, S. Über die sogennanten abnormen Sehnenfäden des Herzens. *Beitr z path Anat u z allg Path* 1906;39:563–584.

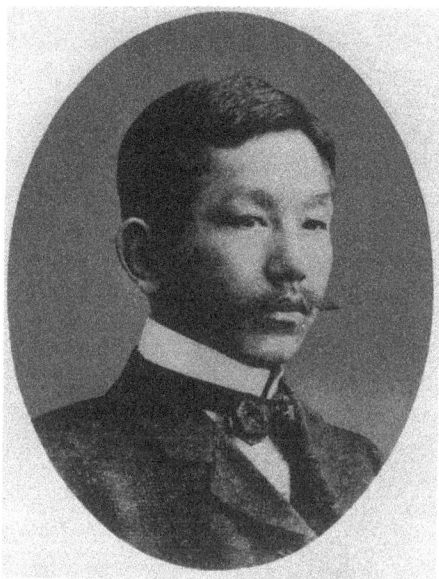

Sunao Tawara (1873–1952)

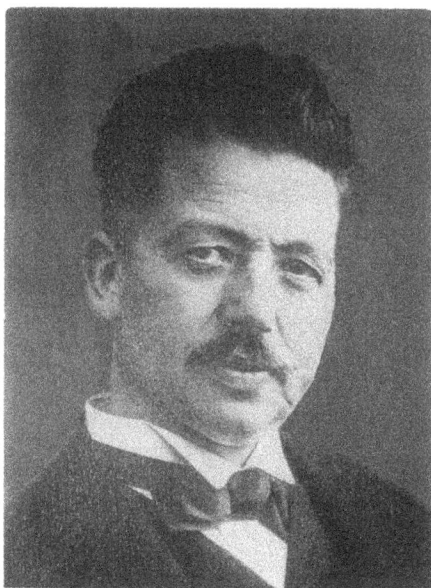

Ludwig Aschoff (1866–1942)

Foreword

I would like to add a few words to the work of Dr. Tawara which follows. The work is the outcome of a systematic investigation using many human and animal hearts and has consumed an enormous amount of time and energy. In this respect, we must also acknowledge the important previous studies of the Leipzig school, spearheaded by Krehl, His and Romberg, since these works gave us the stimulus to reinvestigate both normal and pathological heart specimens.

The increasing attention paid to the value of functional diagnostics in clinical medicine, coupled with the inability of pathologists always to detect a morphological basis for the functional changes in organs, even using the most modern of techniques, has meant that less appreciation is now given to the morphological investigation, a process which was formerly considered essential for understanding the pathological changes. In the light of this situation, it is not without hesitation that a pathologist undertakes the investigation of histological change so as to explain abnormal cardiac activities. As is often the case, nonetheless, it soon became evident in the present study that the thorough investigation of the normal anatomy and histology of the heart was fundamental for the provision of fruitful results.

The extensive investigation of myocarditis I reported briefly at the Congress of the German Association for Pathology at Breslau in 1904 soon made it clear that ignorance in comparing pathological changes with normal findings could lead to serious mistakes. The description by Dr. Tawara which follows indicates that a predominance of sarcoplasm over fibrils, together with the appearance of vacuoles in the sarcoplasm (changes regarded by many authors as partly progressive and partly regressive nutritional disturbances), is an entirely normal phenomenon in a certain kinds of cardiac muscle fibers. It also indicates that various patterns of the nuclei, regarded by many as important evidence for pathological change, do not always indicate abnormality, since such forms of nuclei are not rare even in the normal situation, and it is extremely difficult to demonstrate whether the number of the nuclei is increased under pathological conditions.

The much more important finding of Dr. Tawara than these histological characteristics of the normal cardiac muscle, however, is the following. The connecting bundle discovered by His does not connect the atrial muscle directly with the ventricular muscle, as had previously been thought. Rather, after the formation of a complex node just above the atrioventricular fibrous septum, the bundle penetrates the septum, descends on both sides of the ventricular septum in two discrete bundle branches, and extends into the ventricular cavity through the trabeculations or false tendinous fibers finally to connect with the ventricular musculature in the form of Purkinje fibers at the sites of the papillary muscles and peripheral ventricular layers.

Therefore, I think, a new question arises concerning the physiology of the heart, together with a new concept concerning the relationship between the cardiac chambers. If we admit, on the basis of Hering's experiments which transected the connecting bundle, that normal rhythmical ventricular contractions are generated by excitation originating at the orifice of the superior caval vein and thence conducted through the bundle to the ventricle, then we must conclude from Tawara's findings that the excitation is initially and exclusively transmitted not to the ventricular septal musculature, but through the pathways of almost identical length to all the ventricular components. Furthermore, the impulse probably arrives slightly earlier at the papillary muscles and a little later at the base of the heart. Such a conclusion apparently contradicts the observation of many authors that it is the base of mammalian hearts which is the seat of primary excitation. I would like to emphasize, nonetheless, that the ventricles are originally a fold of an embryological tube and, therefore, that the ventricles are separated into two different parts, namely the posterior part directed toward the venous orifices and the anterior part directed toward the great arteries. This ventricular architecture is not suitable for a simple wave movement of contraction from the base to the apex. The description of the anatomical structure of the heart given in the extensive work of Albrecht, which appeared during our investigation, also supports the opinion of Hesse, Krehl and Braun, nesessarily leading us to recognize the importance of distinguishing the area of the papillary muscles from that of the outflow tracts in each ventricle. The papillary muscles ensure satisfactory closure of the atrioventricular valves by their contraction. The outflow tract is a hollow channel in the left ventricle, and the muscular infundibulum in the right ventricle. The pathological–anatomical observations also indicate that the two areas of each ventricle may be subjected independently to disorders. In any case, the ventricles are constructed in such a complicated fashion — both of the ventricular outflow tracts supporting the great arteries are located anteroposteriorly and above the basal segment of the ventricles, while the papillary muscles are closely connected with the apical portions of the ventricles — that it is impossible for cardiac excitation to spread only from the anterior surface or from the apex of the ventricles. Rather, the excitation must be conducted from different and various sites, such as the posterior surfaces, the apices and the anterior surfaces of both the ventricles and so on. The concept accepted by many physiologists, namely that the excitation wave is simply conducted from the venous to the arterial orifices, seems understandable only when there is continuity between the walls of each cardiac chamber. In other words, the concept would be feasible only when the atrial chambers and ventricles were not almost completely separated one from the other by the development of the connective tissue, and also when the atrial chambers and ventricles were not divided by the septal structures into the right and left components. The reality, however, is the opposite. In fact, the muscle apparatus for the atrioventricular valves are located at the apex of each ventricle, and a special conduction system, His bundle with its branches, really exists. So, a question arises: How, from the anatomical standpoint, is the wave of excitation conducted? From the previous theory that the atrium is connected directly with the ventricular septum through His bundle, an assumption was made that the basal area of the ventricles, directed to the venous orifices, was the first site of excitation. However, this assumption is not acceptable, because His' bundle directly enters the anterior part of the ventricular septum. The first site of excitation, therefore, must be in the proximity of the arterial rather than the venous pole of the ventricles. If the excitation should take place initially in the area controlling the atrioventricular valves, His' bundle should not have its ending in the anterior part of the ventricular septum, but should extend further to the papillary muscles by means of a closed pathway. Tawara's study demonstrates that this is indeed the case. As to excitation, it will be necessary in the future to examine the various segments of the ventricle with more precision than has been achieved before, and such results must be analyzed taking into account the anatomical structure of the conduction pathway.

I would like to emphasize one additional point. H. E. Hering's detailed analysis of the intrinsic rhythm of the human heart indicated that, as shown in the animal experiments, a pacemaker may wander. Sometimes the pacemaker is at its normal location, sometimes it is at the atrioventricular junction, and sometimes it is even inside the ventricle. It was natural, therefore, to regard His bundle as a likely candidate for a hererotopic pacemaker in the conduction system. As Hering stated, any point in the conduction system must be capable of becoming a pacemaker. If this is the reality, then it should be admitted that the special system of muscle fibers ought to have a certain histological difference from the ordinary myocardial fibers. The evidence for this fact is now given for the first time by Tawara's study, together with the old description by Gaskell and Engelmann. This difference is demonstrated most clearly in the hearts of ungulates. In these animals, the whole conduction system is characterized by prevalence of sarcoplasm and reduction of myofibrils. The muscle fibers of the conduction system may be regarded as intermediate in structure between smooth muscle and cross-striated muscle. As a consequence, the hypothesis of Straub that smooth muscle is characterized especially by its rhythmical contraction upon stretching can also be applied to the muscle fibers of the conduction system. As there is no evidence thus far to suggest that the ventricular muscles, from which Purkinje fibers are insulated, move rhythmically by themselves either totally or partially, and since all are suggesting that only the conduction system is the source of heterotopic impulse formation in the heart, I believe that I can give to this system the name of "excitation center," or "cardiomotor center." I do not hesitate to abandon my idea, however, simply because Hering is against me. He insists that automatic excitation usually originates only at one pole. It is then conducted through the remaining system, the other part of the conduction system only exceptionally generating the excitation. I am not yet fully convinced that, in mammalian animals, the initial excitation originates at the junction between the superior caval vein and the right atrium, rather than at the site of so-called "node." I do admit, however, that Hering's analysis corresponds with his view. We will be able to determine the exact location of original excitation of the mammalian heart only when the conduction system, especially the node, is destroyed either by surgery or by thermocauterization. If the atrial contraction remains the same as before, even after destruction of the node, there would be no other possibility than that, in keeping with the presently dominant assumption, automatic excitation originates at the venoatrial junction. At any rate, such an experiment will be of further interest in confirming the significance of the node as a highly complicated structure, known in ungulates also to have a rich nerve supply.

Finally, in this respect, I would like to emphasize that Tawara's study has demonstrated that a great number of nerve bundles accompany the conduction system, at least in ungulates, and that even ganglion cells are scattered within the system. These findings raise new questions. I am convinced, therefore, that I can present Tawara's study to my colleagues with clear conscience for kind verification, despite its breadth of representation, which is contingent on the method of investigation used.

Ludwig Aschoff
Marburg; March 19, 1906

Introduction

In response to a suggestion by Prof. Aschoff, I examined numerous human heart specimens over a period of two-and-a-half years, using the method[1] described by Krehl together with other modern histological staining procedures. I soon realized that the cause of failure of a hypertrophied heart with valvar disease was not yet clearly delineated, although it had been reported that interstitial or parenchymatous lesions might occur in hypertrophied heart muscles. Even the elaborate study by E. Albrecht[2] failed to elucidate the cause of heart failure. I will not discuss here why I cannot accept his pathological and histological explanations, but I will just refer to the preliminary report,[3] which summarized the up-to-then-available results of my studies, presented at the 76th Meeting of the Society of German Natural Scientists and Physicians,[*] held at Breslau. Because the cause of heart failure was not ascribed to histological changes in the cardiac muscle fibers, Prof. Aschoff suggested that I perform an anatomical study of the atrioventricular bundle, to which experimental physiologists, but not anatomists, had given attention.

We began our study with the expectation that pathological changes in the bundle might provide a key to explanation of the disparity between clinical and histological findings regarding valvar heart disease. We soon experienced great difficulty, however, because the normal course and histology of the bundle had not been exhaustively studied. It took nearly two years of uninterrupted study to overcome this difficulty. Previous reports

---

[*]Gesellschaft Deutscher Naturforscher und Ärzte.

by Stanley Kent and by His, and subsequent reports by Retzer and by Braeunig, stated coincidentally that the atrioventricular bundle, immediately after penetrating the atrioventricular fibrous septum, was connected with the ventricular septal muscle. Already, at a very early stage of my research, I was quite embarrassed to realize that I had failed to find such a direct connection anywhere in the ventricular septum. I attempted, therefore, to delineate the whole course of the connecting bundle by examining microscopically numerous serial sections of the bundle.

After conducting time-consuming and energy-wasting examinations for a long period, I finally succeeded in detecting the regularity of the whole course of the bundle. I discovered that Purkinje fibers were the terminal ramifications of the connecting system in human and other animal hearts. I was already convinced of the discovery by the findings relating to the sheep hearts. Although Purkinje fibers were known to exist in certain animal hearts, their function was not clear. My study, therefore, turned into a different direction.

In the following chapters, I will describe the systematic arrangement of the connecting bundle in the human and other animal hearts as accurately as possible. I was forced to limit my investigation to the hearts of humans, dogs, sheep, calves, cats, rabbits and pigeons, because the study was extremely time-consuming. I believe that I have clearly demonstrated the coincidence of the architecture of the connecting system in higher animals and in humans as well as the significant variations among the animal species. I will first describe the precise topography of the system, and then discuss the histological characteristics of the system in each animal species. Thereafter, I will review critically the previous viewpoints concerning Purkinje fibers. Finally, I will summarize my findings regarding the anatomy of the connecting system and its physiological significance.

Because I intend, for the first time in medical history, to propose an integral and consistent explanation concerning the atrioventricular bundle and the Purkinje fibers, I wish to ask your indulgence when I begin by summarizing once again the presently available literature relating to this field.

Hence, before demonstrating the results of my topographical study regarding the atrioventricular connecting bundle, I will begin by reviewing briefly the history of previous investigations concerning the connecting bundle.

A. History

The question as to the existence of a muscular connection between the atrium and the ventricle is so important for understanding cardiac physiology that many studies have already been performed to prove histologically the existence of such a connection.

In v. Kölliker's handbook of histology, and in other works, there are statements that G. Paladino was the first to refer to such a muscular connection. Although I have not been able to find his original paper,[4] I was able to refer to the detailed citation by Boll that appeared in the *Central Journal of Medical Sciences* in 1877. According to Boll's citation, muscle fibers enter the heart valves from both the atrium and the ventricle and, in mammalian hearts, the well-developed atrial muscles enter radially the valves. Indeed, one might mistake tendinous fibers for the continuation of the muscles. I do not intend to discuss here whether the muscle fibers are a part of the valves. I will simply refer to the comprehensive study of E. Albrecht. Even taking Boll's citation into account, nonetheless, I would rather support Retzer, who doubted that Paladino had truly found the direct muscular connection between the atrium and the ventricle. Furthermore, I think that Bardeleben's[5] paper contains an error.

Gaskell[6] was the first to describe exactly the presence of the muscular connections between the heart chambers of cold-blooded animals. He confirmed that, at the borders between the sinus and auricles as well as between the auricles and the ventricles, the net-like arranged muscular tissue joins together to form parallel bundles which are arranged in a ring shape. The ordinary auricular and ventricular muscle tissues originate

3

from the parallel bundles. He concluded from his study that contraction waves are conducted not through the remote nervous apparatus but directly through the muscular tissues from one chamber to the other. He also assumed that the conduction delay at the borders of individual heart chambers was due to different histological characteristics of the muscle fibers in the borders. Gaskell considered that the muscle fibers at the borders are the endings of the ordinary muscle fibers, because they were markedly thin compared with the ordinary ventricular or atrial muscle fibers, and because they had unprominent cross-striations, contained conspicuously abundant and large nuclei, and tapered distally. They were similar structurally to the muscle fibers in the sinus region, where tapering of the fibers is much more prominent. We will see later that Gaskell made important suggestions as to the histological features of the muscular system of the conduction pathway.

Later, A. F. Stanley Kent[7] studied the hearts of rats, guinea-pigs, rabbits and monkeys, and asserted that direct connections were present at the outer margin of the ventricles as well as at the auriculo-ventricular septum between the auricular and ventricular musculatures. He also stated that, even in newborn rats, the muscle fibers in the coronary groove were different from the ordinary cardiac muscle fibers because the former showed a spindle form, and that direct connections between the auricular and ventricular fibers remained lifelong at certain places in the coronary groove and the septum, although the peculiar muscle fibers were reduced by the development of rich connective tissues during the course of somatic growth. According to him, the auriculo-ventricular muscular connections were characterized by networks of fine and ramified muscle fibers, frequently buried in connective tissues in older rats and other animals, especially monkeys. In addition, he stated that these muscle fibers were intermediate between the smooth muscle and the cross-striated muscle through their spindle form and less apparent cross-striations, and that both the auricular and ventricular musculature connected with these characteristic muscle fibers, while the ordinary cardiac muscle fibers split into the network. The histological results described by Kent coincide in several respects with my observation. In contrast, however, I found the connecting bundle only at the junction between the atrial and the ventricular septum, and nowhere in the atrioventricular grooves.

His Jr.[8] discovered the atrioventricular bundle in the human and other mammalian hearts. He indicated in his manuscript entitled "Embryonic Heart Activity and Its Significance for the Theory of Adult Human Heart Action" that a muscular connection existed between the atrial and ventricular chambers in the early developmental stage — even in the embryonic stage — in mammals, and that the initial cardiac contractions occurred prior to the appearance of ganglion cells. It was suggested that excitation was conducted through the muscular system in adult mammals. This idea seems to contradict the generally accepted view that the cardiac muscular tube is interrupted by connective tissue at the atrioventricular margin in mammals, but not in lower animals. His Jr. proved that interruption by the connective tissue was not complete, but rather that a muscular atrioventricular connection existed at a certain location within the atrioventricular fibrous septum. His description was as follows: "After many investigations, I eventually was able to find a muscle bundle which connects the atrial and ventricular septa. This bundle had not been detected previously because it can only be identified when the septal wall is sectioned exactly in the plane of its long axis. Using these longitudinal serial sections, I was able to recognize the course of the bundle in an adult mouse, a newborn dog, two newborn humans, and a 30-year-old-or-so human. The bundle originates at the posterior right atrial wall near the atrial septum above the atrioventricular groove, passes over the upper margin of the ventricular septal muscle, exchanging their fibers manifoldly with each other. It then bifurcates near the aorta into a right and a left bundle branch, the latter terminating at the base of the aortic leaflet of the mitral valve."

In 1904, R. Retzer[9] published a study of the atrioventricular bundle, using the hearts of cats, rabbits, rats, dogs and humans. His report included the following: "The atrioventricular bundle lies just below the membranous part of the ventricular septum, courses backward to the atrial septum and fuses, as His described, with the atrial septal muscle before it reaches the posterior wall of the atrium. It can easily be traced anteriorly, but the situation here is not always the same. The bundle is sometimes situated on the muscular part of the ventricular septum, bifurcates into the right and left branches, and then joins gradually with the ventricular musculature as seen in the atrium. In some microscopical sections, the bundle lies toward the left side of the ventricular septum, spreads widely surrounded by connective tissues, and goes gradually downward. The bundle of muscle fibers becomes gradually thinner until it finally disappears, but clearly seems to combine sequentially with the ventricular muscle fibers." Retzer demonstrated the distinctive histological finding that the atrioventricular bundle was stained somewhat differently than the remaining cardiac musculature, depending upon the direction of the section. He stated: "When the tissue was stained by Haemalaun-Erythrosin, I was unable to find any histological differences from the other muscle fiber, except that the bundle was looser than the other cardiac musculature. Therefore, I could not confirm Kent's statement that the special muscle fibers situated between the atrium and the ventricle are of embryonic origin." It is important to note, however, that he believed he was able to find the course of the bundle macroscopically in one adult human. In one case, he found that the connecting bundle bifurcated into the right and left bundle branches. He estimated the size of the bundle in the adult human heart to be 18 mm long, 2.5 mm wide and 1.5 mm thick. He did not, nonetheless, examine the human heart histologically.

Almost at the same time as the study of Retzer, Braeunig[10] investigated the hearts of a newt, a frog, a ring snake, a young rat and a young lion, two baboon hearts and one human heart. Of special interest are his results regarding the human and mammalian hearts. He stated: "A muscle bundle originates beneath the oval fossa at the right side of the atrial septum, penetrates into the connective tissue between the atrial and ventricular septal structures, and eventually connects directly with the ventricular septal muscle below the membranous septum." He also stated that the connecting muscle fibers and the ventricular muscle fibers are connected beneath the endocardial layer on the left side of the ventricular septum. Further, he recognized that the atrioventricular bundle divides into two branches, and that the upper branch cannot be observed far in the serial sections because it soon fuses completely with the ventricular musculature. In addition, he noted the special staining properties of the atrioventricular bundle, which were caused by its various fiber directions, a loose structure, and the fine connective tissues appearing sporadically between the fibers of the bundle, as shown by Retzer. Braeunig, emphasizing that there was no essential difference between the two types of fibers, said:

"Both longitudinal sections and cross-sections, showing a characteristic polygonal form and central nucleus as demonstrated in Fig. 8, Table I, did not indicate any significant difference between the connecting bundle and the ordinary cardiac musculature." He estimated that the greatest diameter of the bundle surrounded completely by the connective tissue was about 1 mm in a three-to-four-year-old child.

Recently, Max Humblet examined the heart of a dog and also confirmed a muscular connection in the septum. He stated that the muscle fibers of the atrioventricular bundle are thinner than the ordinary cardiac muscle fibers. Macroscopic and microscopic descriptions of only one dog heart, however, are not enough to substantiate this conclusion.

My own study was already considerably advanced when the articles of Retzer and Braeunig were published. Because my findings differed from theirs in many ways, I reported briefly some results in the *Central Journal for Physiology* Vol. 19, No. 3. Prof. Aschoff also presented a summary of the most important microscopical findings at the Congress of Physiology held in Marburg. Thereafter, I re-examined and elaborated the anatomy of the atrioventricular bundle of mammalian hearts more precisely and extensively. This merely reconfirmed the validity of my results that had been presented at the congress held in Marburg. The results will be shown in the following presentation of topographical and histological findings regarding both the human and mammalian hearts.

B. Results of the Study

I. Topography of the Atrioventricular Connecting System

(a) *Dog heart*

(1) *No. 120. The three-day-old dog heart*

This small heart was fixed in its entirety in Formol-Müller, and then the lower half of the ventricle was cut away. The upper half of the ventricle, together with the atrium and great arteries, was then hardened in alcohol and embedded in paraffin, and was cut in the frontal plane serially with a thickness of nine microns in the posteroanterior direction. The axis of the heart was positioned as perpendicularly as possible, the ventricular septum being in the sagittal plane. Every sixth section was stained with Haematoxylin and van Gieson.

In examining the sections, the atrioventricular fibrous septum (*s*) appears in section No. 27 in the form of an arch extending from the site of attachment of the ventricular surface of the leaflet of the mitral valve (*m*) to that of the ventricular surface of the septal leaflet of the tricuspid valve (*t*), the concave side of the arch being directed toward the atrium. Atrial muscle fibers (*v*) located close to the fibrous septum run in parallel with it, and the right side of the atrial muscle mass protrudes toward the broad base of the septal leaflet of the tricuspid valve, taking the shape of a thick tongue (*a*). Left-anteriorly, the protrusion was separated from the ventricular musculature by the fibrous septum and, to the right, from a

8

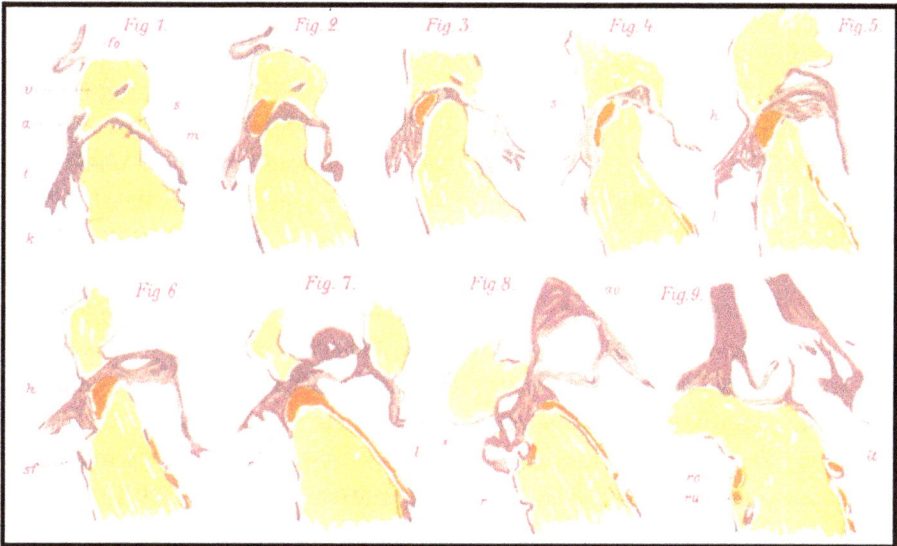

Dog heart No. 120

fo = the oval fossa

v = musculature of the atrial septum

a = tonguelike process of the atrial musculature (see text)

s = the atrioventricular fibrous septum

m = anterior mitral leaflet

t = septal leaflet of the tricuspid valve

k = the ventricular septum

h = initial portion of the ventricular bundle of the connecting system

sf = a tendinous fiber for the septal leaflet of the tricuspid valve

l & r = the left and the right bundle branch of the connecting system

ao = the aorta

lt = a part of muscle fibers of the left bundle branch entering a tendinous fiber-like cord

ro & ru = the right bundle branch separates into two groups (see text)

thin muscular layer by thin connective tissue originating from the site of attachment of the tricuspid valve. A part of the atrial musculature, the thin muscle layer, extends in the subendocardium to the attachment of the tricuspid valve. The appearance of the tongue-shaped muscle mass (*a*) is the same as that of the adjacent atrial musculature. The ventricular septal muscle fibers (*k*) course vertically downward from the arch-shaped fibrous septum. The atrial musculature is stained somewhat paler and contains smaller numbers of nuclei than the ventricular musculature. There is a copious amount of connective tissue in the atrial musculature (Fig. 1).

In the following sections, the tip of the above-mentioned protrusion of the atrial musculature is penetrated and divided into many smaller projections by connective tissue which, arising from the atrioventricular fibrous septum or from the attachment of the septal leaflet of the tricuspid valve, runs in various directions. The connective tissue becomes much more copious, and these projections eventually disappear as serial sections proceed. Consequently, the protrusion becomes shorter, with its head somewhat thicker. Meanwhile, connective tissue, arising from the base of the tricuspid valve and bordering the tongue-shaped muscle protrusion from the right side, gradually extends in the leftward and superior direction. Therefore, the muscle mass of the protrusion becomes more and more separated from the other atrial musculature, but still remains connected with the atrial musculature in its left superior portion. Inside the musculature there appear many thin strands of connective tissue which are in continuity with the tissue encircling the muscle mass on three sides. As a consequence, the muscle mass is divided into many irregularly oriented but interconnected muscle groups. Fiber directions are quite diverse in each group and, even in the same group, the individual muscle fibers take various directions. They are connected to each other to form a cluster. The tincture is strikingly pale (Fig. 2 = section No. 33).

In sections No. 34 and No. 35, the muscle groups are completely isolated from the ordinary atrial musculature at the left superior portion by a plate of connective tissue which arises from the left half of the atrioventricular fibrous septum and combines with connective tissue originating from the base of the septal leaflet of the tricuspid valve. The isolated muscle fiber groups are now situated in the middle of the right half of the fibrous septum, between the ventricular and the atrial septal musculature, surrounded by connective tissues of the atrioventricular fibrous septum. The shape of the muscle groups as a whole is semilunar, the convex side being directed to the left and inferiorly (Fig. 3 = section No. 35).

In the following series (sections No. 36–38), connective tissue fibers bordering the atrial side of the muscle groups become very thick and form a characterisitic arch-shaped atrioventricular fibrous septum. In other words, the muscle bundle has already shifted into the ventricular septum, but is separated from the ordinary ventricular musculature by a thin connective tissue sheath connected to the fibrous septum at both ends. The muscle bundle is penetrated by many connective tissue fibers and divided into many components (Fig. 4 = section No. 38).

In the next two sections, the muscle bundle becomes slightly larger, taking the shape of a slender half-moon, and takes up its position in the right superior portion of the muscular ventricular septum. The bundle is sharply separated from the ventricular musculature by a connective tissue sheath which is particularly thick at both ends of the muscle bundle. (The diameter of the half-moon cut obliquely is about 1.2 mm, the radius about 0.7 mm, and the thickness of the ventricular septum at this point about 1.2 mm.)

The right inferior tip of the half-moon then extends somewhat inferiorly in sections No. 41 and No. 42. Several slender muscle fiber groups (*l*) now appear far remote from and below the muscle bundle (*h*) under the endocardium of the left side of the ventricular septum. These muscle groups are separated from each other and from the ordinary ventricular musculature (Fig. 5 = section No. 42). The newly appearing subendocardial muscle groups are histologically more similar to the muscle bundle than to the surrounding ordinary ventricular musculature. In the next three sections, the left tip of the bundle extends toward the left, while the right inferior tip extends downward, so that the half-moon becomes somewhat larger. The left-sided subendocardial muscle bundles gradually become larger, fusing with each other and forming a large, long muscle group (*l*). The uppermost portion of the ordinary ventricular musculature separates these two muscle groups (*h* and *l*) one from the other by coursing upward to the left and reaching directly the endocardium on the left (Fig. 6 = section No. 44).

In the following sections (No. 46–49), the main bundle (*h*) increases in length and width toward the left, and the left subendocardial muscle bundle (*l*) extends steeply upward, so that these two bundles (*h* and *l*) gradually join together into one muscle bundle. The right inferior tip (*r*) of the main bundle (*h*) extends further inferiorly. There are numerous connective tissues dividing it into many groups. Meanwhile, the middle portion (*h*) of the bundle becomes somewhat thicker. The shape of the connecting bundle in the frontal section is now no longer half-mooned but rather a reversed V, its top being very thick. The left bundle branch (*l*) is long, whereas the right bundle branch (*r*) is much thicker and shorter. The connecting bundle covers the summit of the ventricular septal musculature (*km*), and is always separated from the ventricular musculature by connective tissue fibers (Fig. 7 = section No. 48).

The right bundle branch (*r*) then extends rapidly and the connection between the right and the left bundle branch (*h* and *l*) gradually becomes more slender and finally disappears, being replaced by loose connective tissue (*x*) forming the attachment of the septal leaflet of the tricuspid valve. The left bundle branch (*l*) is still connected with the main bundle (*h*), which is pressed upon from the right side by the base of the tricuspid valve and rapidly becomes smaller (sections No. 50 and No. 51). In the next three sections, the right bundle branch (*r*), which is already separated from the main bundle, extends further downward in the subendocardium. The right bundle branch is separated by connective tissue fibers from the ordinary ventricular musculature on the left side, and is penetrated by them in many places. The main bundle (*h*) rapidly decreases in size until, finally, only a somewhat thickened head portion of the left bundle branch remains (Fig. 8 = section No. 52).

In the following sections, the right bundle branch is separated into two divisions. While the subendocardial upper division (*ro*) takes the same position, the smaller inferior division (*ru*), surrounded by connective tissue fibers, gradually becomes smaller, enters the ventricular musculature, goes somewhat inferiorly, and then suddenly takes its course vertically downward. Unfortunately, I was unable to follow the division (*ru*) further, because the lower half of the ventricle had already been removed and, consequently, the further course of the division was outside the microscopic preparation. The upper division of the right bundle branch (*ro*) gradually moves to the right and anteriorly, always staying in the subendocardial layer, and again gradually becomes larger (Fig. 9 = section No. 60). In section No. 68, the upper division (*ro*) takes a fairly prolonged descending course. Penetrated by connective tissue fibers and lymph fissures, the muscle bundle of the division is separated into many groups. In section No. 73, the right bundle branch has shifted downward and the individual muscle fibers run more and more vertically downward along the sectional plane — in other words, parallel to the axis of the heart. It is always separated from the adjacent ventricular musculature by fine connective tissue fibers and wide lymph fissures. The right bundle branch disappeared in the further preparations, never being connected with the ordinary musculature during its observed course.

The left bundle branch was followed easily after section No. 52. Its upper portion is markedly thick, and stays just between the round left superior edge of the ventricular septal musculature and the membranous part of the septum. As most of the muscle fibers at this portion take their courses anteriorly, they are sliced transversely. Beginning from the thickened upper portion, a thin subendocardial muscle layer extends vertically downward and slightly anteriorly (Fig. 8). In the sections which follow, the upper portion of the left bundle branch reduces in size rapidly, and almost disappears in section No. 54. The thin subendocardial muscle layer gradually decreases in size from above. The lower continuation of the muscle layer cannot be determined, because the lower half of the ventricle had been cut off. The left bundle branch, nonetheless, is well recognized even at the lowest margin of every section. The muscle fibers are always separated from the ordinary ventricular musculature by connective tissue.

From section No. 57, niveau of the endocardium is gradually raised at a location approximately 4 mm below the right coronary leaflet of the aortic valve. The elevation becomes conspicuous in the sections which follow, and most of the muscle fibers of the anterior part of the left bundle branch occupy the elevation. The elevation becomes more apparent anteriorly and is consequently recognized as a small trabeculation (Fig. 9, *lt*). The course of the muscle entering the trabeculation cannot be traced, because it is soon outside the preparation. Below the point of appearance of the trabeculation, several small muscle groups of the left bundle branch are seen running downward and anteriorly. These muscle groups enter another smaller trabeculation and leave the subendocardial position. The termination of the muscle groups could not be determined, as I could not follow the left bundle branch any further anteriorly.

It is noteworthy that, outside the above-mentioned pathways of the right and the left bundle branch, I have found muscle fibers in various parts of the ventricular wall which are histologically the same, or appear almost the same, as the fibers of the above-mentioned system. These muscle fibers always lie in the subendocardium. I used the term "muscle fiber" for the sake of simplification. In fact, the system in the dog consists of large pale cells lying one after another and showing sparse longitudinal and cross-striations, not in any way typical of the cardiac muscle fibers. I will describe this appearance more precisely in the chapter devoted to histology. Sometimes many cells lie one upon the other or side by side and look like a multilayered epithelium, whilst other times the cells form only one or two layers.

In summary, the connecting bundle originates from the lowest portion of the atrial septum, penetrates the atrioventricular fibrous septum anteriorly, runs a short distance anteriorly as a compact bundle, and then bifurcates into the right and the left bundle branch. The smaller right bundle branch is divided further downward into two twigs and runs anteroinferiorly surrounded by connective tissue fibers. The left bundle branch, wide from the beginning, becomes wider downward and is divided into different groups, parts of which enter the trabeculations. It is important to note that the muscle fibers of both the bundle branches never connected with the ordinary cardiac muscle fibers within the lowest margins of the preparations — in other words, approximately to the mid portion of the ventricles.

(2) *In addition to the heart of the three-day-old dog (No. 120) which I have described precisely above, four hearts of young dogs were cut in series parallel to the longitudinal axis:*

No. 119 (3-day-old), from the left to the right;
No. 121 (9-day-old), from the right anterior to the left posterior;
No. 129 (1.5-day-old), anteroposteriorly;
No. 133 (1.5-hour-old), from the right to the left.

These hearts were fixed and stained in the same way as for heart No. 120, and then cut in series in the directions listed above. At this time, I did not have any doubt about the existence of the connecting bundle, but I wanted to make sure of its exact course. I thought that clarification of the exact course of the connecting bundle was essential for finding pathological changes, if any, in human hearts. Contrary to my expectations, however, the direction of the sections was not suitable for clarifying the exact course of the connecting bundle.

In all these hearts, I always found without any exception the atrial segment of the connecting bundle, the characteristic connecting bundle between the atrial and ventricular septal muscles, and its bifurcation into the bundle branches. I could not clarify in these specimens, however, where and how the connecting bundle originated and terminated. What I could confirm from these sections was the fact that the muscle fibers of the connecting bundle do not connect immediately to the ventricular muscle as all previous investigators have stated up to now, but the muscle fibers were always able to be followed at least as far as the middle portion of the ventricular septum as closed bundle branches on both sides of the ventricular septum. The left bundle branch was wide in all specimens and became wider and thinner downward, splitting into various groups. On the other hand, the right bundle branch was small and round from the beginning, gradually becoming much smaller distally. In one specimen, as in No. 120, the right bundle branch was divided into two twigs in its upper course, but they joined together again after a short distance.

In addition, besides both the bundle branches, I noticed subendocardial cell groups or cell cords scattered here and there which looked histologically the same as the cells of the bundle branches. I will describe these findings later in detail. I tried to find the relationship between these scattered cell groups and one of the branches of the connecting bundle, but could not find any direct connections. Thus, the course of the connecting bundle, which was unclear anyway, became even more difficult to understand. Particularly, I could not explain for the time being the nature of these scattered cell groups, which contrasted histologically so sharply with the ordinary cardiac musculature.

Further, I examined in these preparations all the other atrioventricular junctional regions, namely the atrioventricular grooves in addition to the cardiac septum, and searched for the connecting fibers. Stanley Kent described in his study that connecting fibers existed in young and adult animals in abundance between the left atrial and left ventricular parietal walls, as well as between the right atrial and right ventricular parietal walls. According to his description, the connecting fibers run almost vertically from the atrial to the ventricular wall. The connecting fibers should, therefore, be seen longitudinally in my sections and ought easily to be confirmed on examination. In spite of this potentially favorable disposition, coupled with my elaborate investigations, I could not confirm the presence of the connecting fibers which Kent described in any of these five hearts. In all these areas, the atrial musculature was separated from the ventricular musculature by a more or less thick connective tissue layer.

(3) *No. 166. The heart of a big dog*

This specimen was sliced approximately parallel to the line connecting the deepest attachment of the noncoronary and the right coronary aortic leaflet — in other words, horizontally from above to below with the heart in its own upright position. The descriptions are given in the situation of the ventricular septum positioned sagittally. I used terms such as "left," "right," "anterior," "posterior," "superior," "inferior" and so on, therefore, not as really seen under the microscope, but as follows: toward left as though toward the left ventricle; superiorly as though toward the base of the heart; inferiorly as though toward the apex of the heart; anteriorly as though toward the anterior cardiac wall; and so on. In order to understand my directional descriptions correctly, it is important to keep this nomenclature in mind. The nomenclature is also valid in the majority of my other directional descriptions.

In section No. 19, a part of the connecting bundle (x) is seen surrounded by the hard thick aortic fibrocartilaginous connective tissue (s) in the middle of the origin of the aorta. The site of the connecting bundle, when seen from the left ventricle, is approximately in the middle of the noncoronary aortic leaflet, namely 0.7 mm superior to the deepest attachment of the leaflet (Fig. 1 = section No. 19). The bundle becomes rapidly larger in the following sections. It lengthens anteriorly in cuneiform fashion, pushing the thick aortic tissue aside on both sides. Already in section No. 25, it reaches the midpoint between the deepest attachments of the noncoronary and right coronary aortic leaflets. Both the left and the right side of the bundle are bordered by the aortic tissue, and the right aortic tissue is a part of the atrioventricular fibrous septum. In section No. 20, a very small muscle group of the ventricular septum (km) emerges close to the posterior tip of the connecting bundle and very rapidly enlarges in the following sections. It lengthens anteriorly and gradually intrudes in

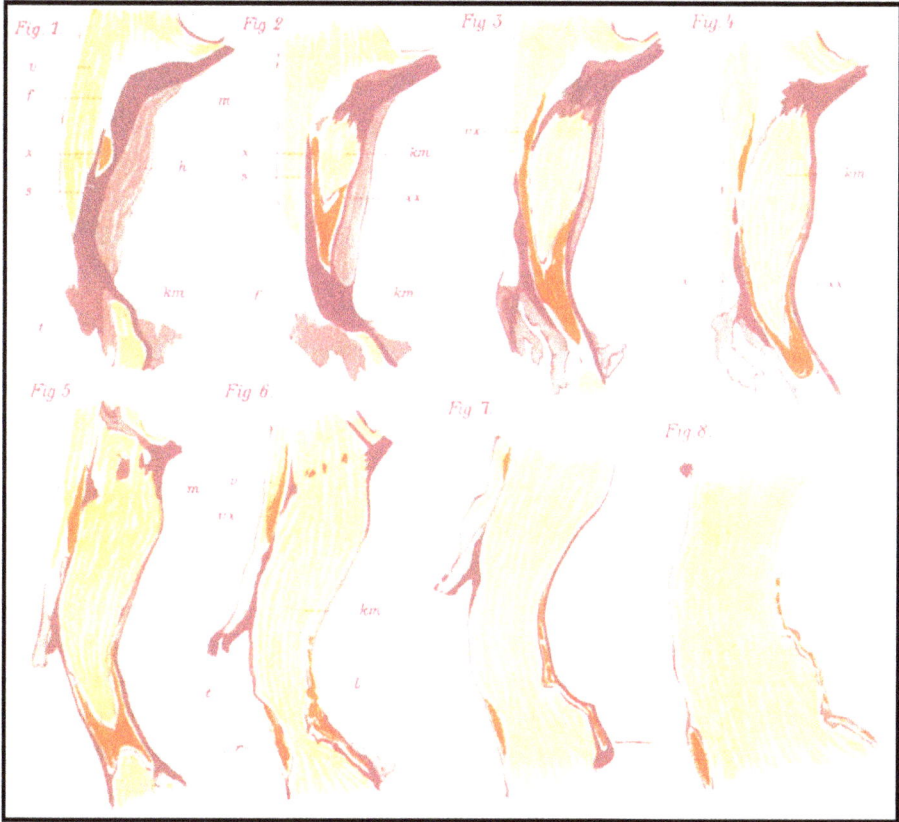

Dog heart No. 166

v, s, m, t, r and l are the same as in the figures for dog heart No. 120.

    x = initial portion of the ventricular bundle

    h = deepest attachment of the noncoronary aortic leaflet

    f = fatty tissue

  km = musculature of the ventricular septum

  vx = atrial segment of the connecting system

  xx = upper portion of the left bundle branch

cuneiform fashion into the bundle posteriorly, so that the posterior tip of the bundle now assumes a fork shape (Fig. 2 = section No. 23). A branch of the fork (*xx*) lies in a thin and long area just posterior to the deepest attachment of the noncoronary aortic leaflet, while the other branch (*x*) is a part of the bundle lying between the ventricular musculature (*km*) and the atrioventricular fibrous septum (*s*).

Up to now, the connecting bundle has not been seen in the atrium. The left side of the atrioventricular fibrous septum is bordered by fatty tissue (*f*), which occupies a long and wide area of the middle portion of the atrial septum. In section No. 25, the connecting bundle lengthens posteriorly and breaks through the fibrous septum. The posterior part (*vx*) of the bundle extends into the fatty tissue. In the following sections, the posterior extension of the bundle becomes much more evident in the atrium (Fig. 3 = section No. 28). It contains plentiful interstitial connective tissue fibers and numerous nuclei, some of which are the nuclei of the connective tissue fibers. Here, the individual muscle fibers run irregularly in various directions, connect very obviously with each other, and form a thick complicated network, which is completely different from the formation of the networks of the ordinary cardiac muscle fibers. By its several peculiarities, the bundle is easily differentiated from the ordinary atrial musculature. This highly thickened network gradually becomes loose at its posterior tip, and individual muscle fibers run more parallel to the posterior. There is also especially rich connective tissue posteriorly. The network, namely the anterior half of the atrial segment of the connecting bundle, lies between the ventricular and the atrial musculature. It is separated from the ventricular musculature by the relatively thin atrioventricular fibrous septum, and from the atrial musculature by a thin connective tissue layer. The structure is spindle-shaped and its size is about 3.0 × 0.7 mm in this very big dog. Anteriorly, the muscle fibers connect with the initial portion of the ventricular segment of the bundle, in which the muscle fibers are arranged more parallelly. Posteriorly, the muscle fibers of the network extend toward the posterior portion of the atrial segment. There is, however, no distinct boundary between the anterior and the posterior part of the structure. The muscle fibers of the network seem not to connect with the surrounding ordinary atrial muscle fibers at all or, at best, connect very sparsely.

The muscle fibers, however, gradually connect one after another with the ordinary atrial musculature (*v*) at the posterior of the atrial bundle. This connection usually takes place so gradually that it is difficult to determine a boundary. I could follow the atrial segment of the connecting bundle until section No. 46, namely until about 2.3 mm below the deepest attachment of the noncoronary aortic leaflet (Figs. 3–7, *vx*).

Now, I come back to the ventricular segment of the bundle. From section No. 25, the anterior tip very slowly lengthens anteriorly and the above-mentioned ventricular muscle (*km*) also gradually enlarges to extend further anteriorly. Consequently, the fork-shaped bifurcation of the bundle becomes thinner. In section No. 33, the right branch of the fork (*x*), which connects directly with the atrial segment of the bundle (*vx*), is eventually broken by the ventricular musculature and is separated from the atrial segment of the bundle. The size of the left branch of the fork (*xx*) is also gradually reduced from behind (Figs. 3 and 4 = sections No. 28 and No. 31). The anterior tip of the bundle, which formerly extended anteriorly and almost horizontally along the inferior limb of the membranous septum, now reaches its lowest point in sections No. 33 and No. 34. In section No. 34, the bundle is bordered by the conical ventricular musculature (*km*) anteriorly and posteriorly and by the endocardium of the right and the left side of the ventricular septum (Fig. 5 = section No. 35).

In the following sections, the two conical ventricular muscles approach together, eventually join each other and form a continuous muscle mass. The ventricular segment of the connecting bundle is divided into two groups, namely the right (*r*) and the left (*l*) bundle branch. It is now clear that a part of the left branch of the fork is the uppermost portion of the left bundle branch (Fig. 6 = section No. 38).

In the following sections, the left bundle branch (*l*) gradually becomes thinner inferiorly and wider horizontally, spreading further anteriorly in the subendocardium. After separation from the right bundle branch, the width of the left bundle branch is about 6 mm at a level directly beneath the line connecting the lowest attachments of the noncoronary and right coronary aortic leaflets. At the beginning, the left bundle branch has dense interstitial connective tissue. The left bundle branch is separated from the adjacent ventricular musculature by dense connective tissue which is a continuation of the aortic base. The interstitial and the separating connective tissue gradually become more sparse inferiorly (Fig. 7 = section No. 43). The left bundle branch becomes thinner and wider inferiorly. In section No. 60, the horizontal subendocardial width of the left bundle branch is about 10 mm, at a level approximately 4 mm beneath the lowest attachment of the right coronary aortic leaflet. Here, the left bundle branch extends from the anterior one third of the noncoronary leaflet to the posterior two thirds of the right coronary aortic leaflet. Up to now in its course, the left bundle branch has always been separated from the ventricular musculature by relatively thick connective tissue. The individual muscle fibers do not run as tightly nor as parallelly as the adjacent ventricular musculature, but rather as loose bundles running in various directions. The muscle fiber bundles, as well as the individual muscle fibers, have their own relatively thick connective tissue sheaths. The preparation ends at section No. 60, but the left bundle branch has not terminated, and is still represented by a broad and thin bundle. The muscle fibers do not connect with the ventricular musculature (Fig. 8 = section No. 58).

The right bundle branch is as large as the left bundle branch immediately after branching. It rapidly becomes smaller in the following sections and its position moves gradually anteroinferiorly. The individual muscle fibers run closely and parallel to each other. The overall muscle bundle is surrounded by a connective tissue sheath and is sharply separated from the adjacent ventricular musculature. Interstitial connective tissue also exists abundantly within the right bundle branch. In this preparation, the right bundle branch took its course in the subendocardium from the beginning and was easily traced up to the last section.

Everywhere, the connecting bundle was easily differentiated from the ordinary musculature by its histological peculiarities as far as it was identified in the preparation. The histology of the bundle was not always the same but showed significant differences at its various portions. I will describe this point later.

(4) *No. 167. The heart of a big dog*

As the method which was used in preparation No. 166 proved to be the best for studying the course of the connecting bundle, I again made a series of sections as similarly as possible in the big dog heart to confirm the findings described earlier. The findings obtained from this preparation were surprisingly similar on the whole to those from preparation No. 166, apart from several insignificant differences. Nevertheless, it seems necessary for me to describe again these findings with precision, because there has been no detailed description until now of the course of the connecting bundle in a dog, and also because physiological experiments on the connecting bundle are frequently performed using dog hearts — I am concerned, therefore, lest uncertain anatomical knowledge might lead to inadvertent and erroneous conclusions.

On examining this preparation, in section No. 15, for the first time, a small special muscle mass appears immediately posterior to the origin of the aorta. When seen from the left ventricle, it lies in the middle of the posterior half of the noncoronary aortic leaflet and about 1 mm above its lowest attachment, and is separated from the atrial musculature to the right and posteriorly by thick fatty tissue. In the next two sections, this peculiar mass enlarges and intrudes into the strong connective tissue of the aorta. In section No. 18, it breaks through the connective tissue layers and rapidly lengthens anteriorly along the left side of the origin of the aorta, namely between the aortic origin and the lowest point of attachment of the noncoronary aortic leaflet. Ventricular septal musculature now gradually appears posterior to the above-mentioned muscle mass.

In the following sections, the connecting muscle bundle lengthens further not only anteriorly but also posteriorly. In section No. 23, it finally connects posteriorly with the ordinary atrial musculature. It also extends anteriorly with its round tip into the thick connective tissue at the origin of the aorta and reaches the mid-point between the noncoronary and right coronary aortic leaflets. The above-mentioned ventricular septal musculature enlarges and shows a beautiful oval shape in the following sections. It borders the posterior portion of the connecting bundle from the left. There is no connection, however, between the two kinds of muscle; they are sharply separated by connective tissue. The size of the connecting bundle at the point of the breakthrough at the origin of the aorta, which is a portion of the atrioventricular fibrous septum, is about 1 mm (up to section No. 23).

In the following sections, the oval ventricular muscle enlarges further and the right side of the muscle reaches the thick connective tissue of the origin of the aorta, this representing the atrioventricular fibrous septum. Consequently, the connecting bundle is divided into two segments: the atrial and the ventricular.

First of all, I will describe the atrial segment of the connecting bundle. From section No. 23, it gradually becomes longer posteriorly and connects extensively with the atrial musculature, especially to the right and posteriorly. Its left side, however, is bordered by fatty tissue. Only at the posterior portion do several muscle fibers of the connecting bundle, after running through the fatty tissue, connect with the ordinary atrial musculature at the left half of the septum. In sections No. 26 and No. 27, the atrial segment shows its greatest horizontal width, of about 0.9 mm. Then it slowly becomes thinner again. It lengthens further posteriorly, however, until it reaches its greatest length (about 5 mm) in sections No. 30 and No. 31. As the section numbers progress, the atrial segment rapidly becomes thinner and the number of muscle fibers is reduced, especially at its posterior portion, with larger gaps appearing between them. The gaps are filled either with connective tissue fibers or with fatty tissue. On the other hand, its anterior portion remains thick and maintains its spindle form. It rapidly becomes smaller until it finally disappears in section No. 50. The shape of the atrial segment of the connecting bundle in this specimen is a spindle. It can easily be differentiated from the adjacent atrial musculature using a magnifying glass because of its thickness and compactness, while the atrial musculature, mostly sectioned transversely, is divided into fields, and interconnecting narrow gaps are recognized giving the appearance of a net. The connecting bundle is stained red–brown, whereas the atrial musculature is stained yellow–brown. This difference is due to the fact that the connecting bundle apparently contains many connective tissue fibers which are stained bright red by van Gieson stain. Using stronger magnification, the difference between the connecting bundle and the ordinary atrial musculature is more apparent because the histological appearance and the arrangement of the muscle fibers of the connecting bundle are so peculiar. The complicated plexus-like arrangement of the muscle fibers in the anterior portion of the atrial segment is especially distinct in this heart, as described previously for preparation No. 166.

After penetrating the atrioventricular fibrous septum, i.e. the thick connective tissue of the aortic base, the initial portion of the ventricular segment of the connecting bundle appears at the most posterior margin of the noncoronary aortic leaflet, approximately at the height of the lowest attachment, as already mentioned. It runs horizontally and anteriorly along the left margin of the fibrous septum. The most anterior tip reaches the point where the noncoronary and right coronary aortic leaflets meet. During its course, the bundle gradually becomes wider anteriorly in the horizontal plane. The anterior part of the bundle covers the top of the ordinary ventricular septal musculature from above, while the posterior part runs through a channel between the atrioventricular fibrous septum and the top of the ventricular musculature. The widest place of the ventricular segment of the bundle, namely the most anterior tip, is about 1.8 mm. There is a shallow groove at the lower surface of this wide anterior part of the bundle into which the top of the ventricular musculature is inserted. Thus, the ventricular musculature is covered with the connecting bundle (sections No. 18–30).

After reaching the anterior portion of the noncoronary aortic leaflet, the connecting bundle suddenly turns inferiorly and slightly anteriorly. In sections No. 32–34, it is gradually divided into two portions, namely the left and the right bundle branch. Each bundle branch lies directly under the left-side and the right-side endocardium of the ventricular septum, respectively. The two bundles are separated by the ventricular musculature. In other words, the ventricular segment of the connecting bundle straddles the septal crest with its two bundle branches. The length of the ventricular segment of the connecting bundle from its beginning to the point of branching in this specimen is about 9 mm.

The left bundle branch, containing less muscle fibers than the right, takes its subendocardial course almost vertically downward and somewhat anteriorly. The fibers are separated by a connective tissue sheath, which can be seen even under weak magnification. Individual muscle fibers usually run parallel to the direction of the bundle branch. They are, therefore, mostly sectioned obliquely or transversely. The width of the branch is approximately 4 mm and the thickness is minimal. The width decreases slightly as it descends (for example, about 3 mm in section No. 57) and then increases again further below. The number of the fibers in the left bundle branch increases slightly downward, but remains almost constant. Up to now, the left bundle branch has been separated from the ordinary ventricular musculature by a connective tissue sheath, and nowhere do the fibers of the branch connect with the ordinary ventricular musculature. This preparation ended about 3.5 mm below the aortic valve.

The right bundle branch is relatively large at its origin in this specimen, and is sectioned as a beautiful oval shape. It runs inferiorly and anteriorly in the subendocardial layer. Gradually the cross-section becomes longer. Passing close to the small medial papillary muscle, the right bundle branch runs almost horizontally and anteriorly and goes outside the preparation in section No. 50. The right bundle branch was always surrounded with a thin connective tissue sheath and the muscle fibers during their course never connected with the adjacent ventricular musculature.

From the two preparations described precisely above (hearts No. 166 and No. 167), we have learned that the proximal portion of the connecting bundle takes a predictable course, always maintaining a constant relationship with its adjacent tissues, and that the connecting bundle bifurcates into the left and the right bundle branch in all specimens. It is not clear, however, how far and in what condition the two bundle branches go before they reach their ends. In order to solve this problem, I made further studies of the left and the right bundle branch using dog hearts.

(5) *No. 157. The heart of a medium-sized adult dog*

This specimen was used exclusively for the study of the left bundle branch of the connecting bundle. Only horizontal sections of the left ventricle were made, therefore, from the base to the apex. To make the specimen as small as possible, the peripheral portion of the free wall and the right half of the septum were cut away in advance (compare with procedures for cat and sheep hearts).

In this specimen, the left bundle branch of the connecting bundle is recognizable immediately from the first section by its histological characteristics. It lies in the subendocardium beneath the line connecting the lowest attachments of the noncoronary and right coronary aortic leaflets. The horizontal width is about 3 mm and it is very thin, usually only several fibers thick. The bundle branch is separated from the adjacent ventricular musculature by connective tissue, and there is much connective tissue between the muscle fibers, which are mostly sectioned transversely and occasionally obliquely. When this bundle is followed further downward, it gradually broadens anteriorly and posteriorly as it descends. In its upper course, the bundle is divided into two or three groups by subendocardial connective tissue, but they soon join together. It divides again, however, about 5 mm beneath the aortic leaflets, into two groups (A and B), and further below into three groups (C). The three muscle groups gradually separate from each other as they go down. The most anterior group (A) goes antero-obliquely, the majority of the fibers finally leaving the subendocardial layer of the ventricular septum and entering a small trabeculation covered with an endocardial layer, a so-called false tendinous fiber.[*] In contrast, the other fibers of the group run further downward in the subendocardial layer and split into many small muscle groups. Some of the groups again run into thin connective tissue cords, leaving the septum. The posterior muscle group (C) runs downward and somewhat posteriorly, and is itself divided into two groups which enter false tendinous fibers. The middle muscle group (B) similarly enters a false tendinous fiber. Only a few muscle fibers still remain in the subendocardial layer and take their courses further downward. All the false tendinous fibers containing the muscle fibers of the left bundle branch run downward in the ventricular cavity for a variable distance, divide themselves into several branches, and combine with other branches of the false tendinous fibers. Consequently, they constitute a gross network in the ventricular cavity. Most of the cords and their branches attach to the anterior and the posterior papillary muscle. The other cords and their branches attach to the lower one-third of the ventricular wall. From all the attachments, the muscle fibers of the connecting bundle spread in various directions in the subendocardium, mostly in narrow bands but occasionally in wide bands. The direction of the individual muscle fibers of the left bundle branch is mostly vertically downward in the beginning but it becomes gradually haphazard, with some of the fibers not infrequently running horizontal.

When other sections are examined, directly beneath the endocardium even at the uppermost portion of the posterior septal wall, special muscle

---

[*]*falscher Sehnenfaden*

fibers can be seen, separated from the adjacent ventricular musculature by connective tissue. These muscle fibers, lying scattered within subendocardial connective tissue, are histologically similar to the ordinary left ventricular muscle fibers. The former, nonetheless, seems to have no relationship with the latter. When the muscle groups are more precisely followed, they enter a small short false tendinous fiber and go to the neighboring wall, spreading here again as a broad thin layer in the subendocardium. In addition to the muscle groups already mentioned, other muscle groups, either narrow or broad, appear in the subendocardium at different parts of the wall. Because of their countless number and of their irregular form, and because histological differences are insufficient to distinguish them from the adjacent ventricular muscle fibers, it is often difficult to follow these individual groups. Nevertheless, by exhaustive examinations, the subtle characteristic architecture and the abundant connective tissue existing not only between the fibers, but also between the fibers and the ventricular musculature, made it possible to differentiate the subendocardial muscle groups from the adjacent ventricular musculature. The differentiation, however, was very difficult when only a small amount of connective tissue separated the two kinds of muscle. It was also difficult when there were numerous direct connections between the two. This was, in fact, often the case.

When the subendocardial muscle groups are carefully followed, it is found that they are not scattered in isolation like islands, but rather have relationships to each other. The relationships are as follows. Sometimes, a small short strand of connective tissue, connecting two portions of the wall like a bridge in the ventricular cavity, transfers several muscle fibers from one muscle group to another. Sometimes, several muscle fibers run in the subendocardium connecting two neighboring muscle groups. And sometimes, a subendocardial muscle group connects directly with a muscle bundle, representing a terminal ramification of the left bundle branch. Those muscle bundles enter many false tendinous fibers as the terminal ramifications and spread in various parts of the wall, especially at the sites of both papillary muscles. I observed most frequently the first type of connection between a papillary muscle and the adjacent ventricular wall and then around the cardiac apex, where numerous trabeculations developed and, accordingly, an unevenness of the wall was prominent. Not infrequently,

I also observed these fine connections at other portions of the wall. *As a consequence, a conclusion can be made that the numerous subendocardially scattered muscle groups are related to each other, and also to the terminal ramifications of the left bundle branch of the connecting bundle. In other words, all of the muscle groups are the terminal ramifications of the connecting bundle.*

In this way, the left bundle branch spreads almost everywhere inside the inner ventricular wall of the dog. In the histological studies of the very young dogs, No. 119, 120, 121, 129 and 130, I have already described that, in many subendocardial areas, there appeared a great number of peculiar, large and vesicular cells which lie closely side by side and one upon the other in two, three or rarely more layers. The cells are histologically quite similar to those of the left or right bundle branch of the connecting bundle, but they seem to bear no relation to the bundle branches. At that time, I could not really explain the significance of these peculiar subendocardial cell groups. I can now conclude with certainty, however, that the peculiar subendocardial cell groups of the small dogs must be the terminal ramifications of the connecting bundle. This is because I have discovered from the findings of specimen No. 157 that the terminal ramifications of the left bundle branch spread almost everywhere beneath the endocardium of the ventricle. Although histologically the cells differ greatly between the small dogs and this specimen, and they do not look similar to each other, the histological difference can easily be explained by the age difference.

In the dog heart, the terminal ramifications of the connecting bundle do not always spread in the form of a fiber, but often in a more or less flat band in the subendocardium. Spreading in the form of a fiber is more usually seen. The terminal ramifications are separated from the ordinary myocardium by variably abundant subendocardial connective tissue. As the muscle fibers run loosely in loose connective tissue, it appears that they lie separately from each other in a connective tissue mesh when sectioned transversely. Abundant connective tissue between the muscle fibers, i.e. the sheath of connective tissue surrounding the muscle fibers, seems to be very characteristic of this system. Otherwise, there are no significant differences between this system and the ordinary ventricular musculature. This will be described later.

The terminal ramifications of the connecting system usually take their courses in a very thin layer in the subendocardium, mostly arranged only one or two fibers thick, rarely more. Sometimes, they run only as a single layer of muscle fibers separated from others by subendocardial connective tissue. They either connect soon with a fiber of the ordinary ventricular musculature or branch after a short distance into two or more fibers. The muscle fibers of the terminal ramifications connect in continuity with the ordinary ventricular musculature at various subendocardial sites. In spite of my efforts to find end points of the terminal ramifications of the system in the myocardium, I could not observe any with certainty in any of the above-mentioned specimens. Nevertheless, it cannot be denied that, as in the sheep and calf, there are intramyocardial terminal ramifications also in the dog. This is because it is possible that, through a further fibrillary differentiation, a fiber forming an intramyocardial terminal ramification might appear very similar to an ordinary myocardial fiber. The similarity would make the exact distinction between the two kinds of fiber very difficult.

(6) *No. 12. The heart of an adult big dog*
Description of the right bundle branch

From the above examinations, we already have a knowledge as to how the right bundle branch divides from the left bundle branch, and how the upper portion takes its course. Its further course, nonetheless, was still obscure. I had, therefore, to make a number of histological specimens of many dog and human hearts until I could orientate the course of the right bundle branch. Preparation No. 12 is one of these specimens. It was made as follows: a part of the right half of the ventricular septum, possibly containing the right bundle branch, was serially sectioned from posterior to anterior, vertical to the septal surface and parallel to the cardiac axis. After the bifurcation of the connecting bundle into the left and the right bundle branch, the right runs more anteriorly and somewhat inferiorly in the ventricular musculature as a closed bundle surrounded by a connective tissue sheath, and soon reaches the endocardium of the right side of the septum. The right bundle branch is divided into many fields by connective tissue. Here, the thickness of the bundle branch is about 0.4 mm. While the main bundle of the right bundle branch runs in the subendocardium more anteriorly and somewhat inferiorly, a part of the bundle again enters the ventricular musculature (section No. 19), running vertically downward and slightly anteriorly. This part of the bundle runs further downward in the ventricular musculature, becoming gradually smaller and approaching the endocardium. It finally joins the main bundle, which always takes its course downward in the subendocardium. The right bundle branch is very thin at this point and individual muscle fibers run more or less vertically downward, almost parallel to the direction of the bundle itself (section No. 51).

Already at the lower end of section No. 30, a peculiar muscle bundle appeared in the subendocardium, being separated from the ordinary ventricular musculature by fatty tissue and connective tissue and containing interfascicular connective tissue. The muscle fibers seem identical to the muscle fibers of the right bundle branch and quite different from the ordinary musculature. In the subsequent sections, the muscle bundle gradually lengthens upward, gradually becomes thinner and finally connects with the major component of the right bundle branch, which is elongating from a superior to inferior direction (section No. 54). In other words, this muscle bundle, which appeared in section No. 30, was nothing but the continuation of the right bundle branch running in a slight arc convexed anteriorly. The right bundle branch is relatively wide (2–3 mm) in its course below the mid point and is very thin, usually only several fibers thick and often with inner gaps.

As a rather wide bundle, the right bundle branch reaches the anterior transition from the ventricular septum to the right ventricular parietal wall. This specimen ended at a level about 2.4 cm below the anterior attachment of the septal leaflet of the tricuspid valve. The termination of the right bundle branch, therefore, was not found in the specimen.

I, therefore, made a second specimen which was a direct inferior continuation of the above-mentioned specimen. This specimen contained the base of the anterior papillary muscle as well as the transition from the ventricular septum to the parietal wall. The anterior papillary muscle was mainly seated upon the ventricular septum, but was partly attached to the parietal wall by a small leg. The transition was rather smooth throughout its entire length (from the infundibulum to the vicinity of the cardiac apex), unlike human specimens in which trabeculations run in various directions. This specimen was sectioned horizontally from above to below, and vertical to the cardiac axis.

Through examining the histological sections, the right bundle branch can again be recognized as a relatively broad subendocardial bundle, with the muscle fibers quite different from the adjacent ventricular musculature. The right bundle branch runs further downward toward the base of the anterior papillary muscle. After reaching the anterior papillary muscle, it divides into two twigs, one of which enters the small leg mentioned above extending from the papillary muscle. This small bridging leg leads the twig to the parietal wall. The other twig gives forth many small branches in the subendocardium at the papillary muscle, and these twigs spread in various directions in the papillary muscle and its surroundings. I was unable to follow all the twigs.

I would like to summarize briefly the course of the right bundle branch once again, as follows. At its beginning, after bifurcating from the left bundle branch, the right bundle branch goes slightly anteroinferiorly and soon reaches the subendocardium of the right side of the septum. Thereafter, it runs further close to the medial papillary muscle. It continues anteroinferiorly, then gradually downward, as a slightly convex arc, and finally reaches the base of the anterior papillary muscle. Here, it divides into many twigs. In addition, in its upper course, the right bundle branch divides into two branches which rejoin after a short distance. In the whole course, from its origin to the anterior papillary muscle, the right bundle branch is always surrounded by a connective tissue sheath which separates the bundle branch from the ordinary ventricular musculature. *I could not find any connection, throughout its entire long course, between the muscle fibers of the right bundle branch and the ventricular septum.*

(7) *No. 163. The heart of a big adult dog*
Macroscopic description of the connecting bundle

In connection with the above-mentioned microscopic findings, I would like to describe macroscopically the atrioventricular connecting bundle of a big dog heart and show how far the system of such a heart can be traced. Unfortunately, I had to abandon my intention of examining a fresh specimen, as such a dog heart was not obtainable.

Many dog hearts, first fixed in Formol-Müller and then preserved in alcohol, were examined and compared. It soon became clear that the macroscopic appearance of the connecting system was not the same in all hearts, but rather showed considerable individual differences. When the hearts are examined precisely and carefully, however, you can clarify macroscopically the overall arrangement of the system in all hearts. Only small differences are demonstrated in the general structure of the system between different hearts. In general, there is an unmistakable regularity, which I will describe later. As an example, the macroscopic findings from one specimen (No. 163) are detailed here.*

When the strongly contracted left ventricle is cut open (in this heart, I opened the left ventricle carefully at its anterior wall from the aortic orifice to the apex between the papillary muscles), numerous well-developed trabeculations can be seen on the inner surface running from the cardiac apex up to the upper flat area beneath the right coronary and the non-coronary leaflet of the aortic valve. The trabeculations subdivide into many smaller ones, which lie closely by each other and interconnect inferiorly, forming nets and meshes. Both the papillary muscles are relatively bulky and fuse with the wall. The endocardium is transparent and shiny. The underlying myocardium can be seen to be grayish brown except at the place where the left bundle branch of the connecting system runs.

Between the noncoronary and the right coronary aortic leaflet, just below the level of the lowest attachments of the leaflets, the endocardium of a width of about 2.5 mm is nontransparent and grayish. The nontransparent area rapidly widens anteriorly and inferiorly. About 3 mm below and at its posterior margin, a nontransparent tendinous fiber-like cord** of about 1.5 mm width is seen running almost vertically downward. The subendo-cardial cord becomes more apparent inferiorly and raises the endocardium slightly to make a fold. Eventually, a greater part of the cord leaves the muscular septum about 1 cm below the aortic leaflet in the form of a

---

*The macroscopic course of the connecting bundle is demonstrated in another dog in Plate II, Fig. 2, and Plate III, Fig. 1.

**_sehnenfadenartiger Strang_

tendinous fiber-like cord which is flat (2 mm wide) initially and becomes round later. This passes through the ventricular cavity and finally attaches to the tip of the posterior papillary muscle. Just below the site of takeoff of the cord, the rest of the left bundle branch still remains in the subendocardium and forms several clearly visible networks. Later, it also leaves the subendocardium as another round tendinous fiber-like cord. This cord passes through the ventricular cavity toward the posterior papillary muscle and attaches to its middle portion, giving forth five twigs which attach to different sites in the middle and inferior thirds of the left ventricular posterior wall.

Several facts are remarkable in this heart: near the site of attachment of the first tendinous fiber-like cord to the posterior papillary muscle, another cord originates and goes upward to the base of the heart through the ventricular cavity. This is divided into five twigs which attach to various parts of the upper and middle thirds of the posterior wall. When the site of insertion of the first tendinous fiber-like cord, and the site of takeoff of the second, are examined at the papillary muscle, it is found that a gray fiber runs subendocardially between the two sites. From this finding, it is evident that part of the connecting bundle runs to the posterior papillary muscle through the first cord, and reaches the upper portion of the posterior wall in continuity through the second tendinous fiber-like cord. This fact is not unique and occurs often in humans and in other animals. I think this finding is very important.

The left bundle branch becomes wider inferiorly, as I described earlier. About 1.3 cm below the right coronary aortic leaflet, at the anterior border of the bundle branch, another cord gradually develops and leaves the ventricular musculature. This cord attaches to the upper portion of the anterior papillary muscle through three twigs. In addition, another twig is sent to the ventricular septum.

The opacity in the course of the left bundle branch gradually decreases downward, and disappears completely about 1.8 cm below the aortic valve. In the lower part of the opaque region, however, two stripes can be seen running anteroinferiorly in the subendocardium. The anterior stripe eventually becomes a small cord and, after running in a short bridge-like course, it is divided into two twigs which attach to a trabeculation. Another stripe, not leaving the subendocardial position, runs to a neighboring trabeculation and disappears.

What I have described concerned the main bundle of the left bundle branch. When the inner surface of the heart is observed carefully, numerous short tendinous fiber-like cords are visible which are of the thickness of a hair or a stickpin. They stretch either from the papillary muscle to the neighboring ventricular wall, or from one trabeculation to another, bridging recesses between them. Furthermore, many scarcely visible subendocardial stripes are just seen, which are usually thin though occasionally relatively wide, at both the papillary muscles. As found microscopically, they extend in various directions as the terminal ramifications from the attachments of the cords. In this dog, I could not find this kind of subendocardial terminal ramifications in other parts of the left ventricular wall.

The right bundle branch was macroscopically easily recognizable in this heart.

When the right ventricle was opened, the septum was arched to the right in a half-spherical manner as a result of the strong left ventricular contraction. The anterior half of the septal surface was relatively smooth while, in the posterior half of the septal surface, there were numerous protrusions and recesses running vertically. In the surface of the parietal wall, there were many trabecular networks with recesses. The recesses mostly ran convergently from the ventricular base to the apex. Three relatively big papillary muscles were observed in this heart in addition to a small medial papillary muscle. The anterior papillary muscle, the biggest among them, had three bases, attaching to the septum with two and to the parietal wall with the remaining one. The medial papillary muscle attached with several bases exclusively to the septum. The posterior papillary muscle attached to the parietal wall with a flat and conelike base.

The right bundle branch was first visible under the endocardium as a blue–gray cord of about 1.5 mm width at the anteroinferior margin of the membranous septum, at several millimeters below the most anterior point of attachment of the septal leaflet of the tricuspid valve. The surrounding area was brownish gray in color. The right bundle branch then gradually extended anteriorly and somewhat inferiorly, close to the posteroinferior base of the small medial papillary muscle lying underneath the supraventricular crest. After running for about 1 cm further, it curved initially gradually downward and then somewhat inferoposteriorly. It eventually reached the middle portion of the anterior papillary muscle after a 2.5 cm course in a mild arch through the base of the papillary muscle. The bundle branch left its subendocardial position and became a strong blue–gray flat tendinous fiber-like cord. This cord soon divided into many branches which inter-connected with one another through short twigs and formed several meshlike networks. One of these twigs, a very short one, again attached to the anterior papillary muscle. Another twig, an about 2.5-cm-long and horsehair-thick cord, attached to one of the bases of the posterior papillary muscle through the ventricular cavity. This cord sent two fine twigs to the parietal wall. All the other twigs of the right bundle branch went from the site of division at the anterior papillary muscle divergently to the parietal wall, at the same time sending many twigs to various trabeculations of the wall. I could not follow each of the terminal ramifications of the right bundle branch. When observed precisely, nonetheless, it was found that a subendocardial fiber extended from the leg of the anterior papillary muscle to the base of the extra-medial papillary muscle and, further, that a short fine fiber extended from the middle portion of the medial papillary muscle to the base of the posterior papillary muscle.

Besides these terminal ramifications of the right bundle branch, many other tendinous fiber-like cords were observed. These were short cords, at best as thick as a stickpin which bridged recesses between two protrusions. Mostly, they bridged between the papillary muscles and the adjacent wall at the posterior transition from the septum to the parietal wall, and not infrequently between the neighboring protrusions of the septum as well as of the parietal wall. Although macroscopically the fine short cords seemed to have no relation to the right bundle branch in the dog hearts, they were nothing but the terminal ramifications of the connecting bundle. I already confirmed this fact microscopically in the left bundle branch of the dog (No. 157) as well as macroscopically and microscopically in the sheep hearts (No. 155 and No. 160) which I will mention later.

Anyone can easily confirm what I have described about the macroscopic findings, which is very difficult to recognize but by no means an illusion. It is concerned with a widely spreading subendocardial network at the anterior half of the parietal wall, where trabecular protrusions are relatively broad, flat and regular. The network is made up of broad components where it seems the endocardium is thickened. The components, appearing somewhat more grayish than the surroundings, run mostly across or along the trabeculations and connect with the other components. When a component encounters a shallow recess on its course, it frequently lifts up the endocardium. When it crosses a relatively wide and deep recess between two trabeculations, however, it does not go into the depths along with the endocardium but bridges the recess as a short cord and goes further as a thin fiber or as a wide component beyond the recess. When a recess is deep but narrow, the component not infrequently bridges the recess as a broad membrane. I could not find this kind of network macroscopically in the left ventricular wall, perhaps due to too strong unevenness of the wall. This certainly also exists in the left ventricle, nonetheless, since I saw a similar finding microscopically in the left ventricle, as I have already described. Microscopically, this network was proved to be a terminal ramification of the left bundle branch. From this fact, I similarly conclude that the subendocardial network in the right ventricle is the terminal ramification of the right bundle branch.

(b) *Human heart*

(1) *No. 136. The two-year-old child heart*

This preparation was the heart of a child who died of scarlet fever. The heart was fixed in its entirety in Formol-Müller solution. After washing, all the parietal walls were cut away. The upper portion of the septum (from the free edge of the noncoronary aortic leaflet) and the lower portion (from a line about 8 mm below the lowest attachment of the noncoronary aortic leaflet) were cut away parallel to the upper horizontal section line. From this approximately 1.2-cm-high specimen, the anterior portion was cut away, from the mid-line of the right coronary aortic leaflet vertical to the horizontal lines. (In this description, the septum was considered to be sagittal, i.e. anteroposteriorly.) Then, from the posterior portion, which consisted exclusively of the atrial septum and the posterior cardiac wall, the latter was also cut away. Thus, the specimen contained all of the atrioventricular fibrous septum, almost all the length of the line of attachment of the septal leaflet of the tricuspid valve, part of the aortic leaflet of the mitral valve, the oval fossa, part of the coronary sinus, the

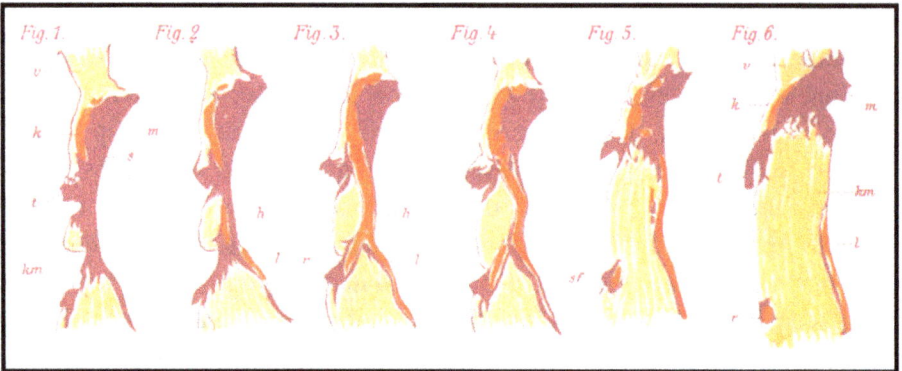

3. Human heart No. 136

> *v*, *m*, *t*, *km*, *s*, *r*, *l* and *sf* are the same as in the figures for dog hearts No. 120 and No. 166.
>
> *k* = node, i.e. atrial segment of the connecting system
>
> *h* = initial portion of the ventricular bundle

membranous septum, the upper portion of the muscular ventricular septum, and so on. Above all, the membranous septum is especially important, because it has already been used by other investigators as a key point with which to describe the course of the atrioventricular bundle. When observed from the left ventricle, the membranous septum, although variable in size, is always found between the right coronary and the noncoronary aortic leaflet, with its lower edge reaching the connecting line between the lowest attachments of both aortic leaflets, or slightly below this level. When seen from the right ventricle, it is found close to the posterior part of the supraventricular crest, namely just at the site where the attachments of the septal and the anterior leaflet of the tricuspid valve join.

This preparation was hardened in high density alcohol, embedded in paraffin, and continuously sectioned horizontally in 12-micron-thick sections, in other words, parallel to the margin of closure of the aortic leaflets and vertical to the cardiac axis. Every fifth section was mounted and stained first with Haematoxylin and then with van Gieson.

By examining the staged microscopic sections, a peculiar muscle group is observed in section No. 105, which is entirely different from the atrial musculature in terms of abundancy and form of nuclei as well as in the arrangement of the muscle fibers. The muscle group is located about 1.5 mm below the lowest attachment of the noncoronary aortic leaflet, in other words, at the inferoposterior margin of the membranous septum. It adheres to the atrioventricular fibrous septum (*s*), i.e. to the origin of the aorta. When compared with the adjacent atrial muscle fibers, the fibers are much smaller and less differentiated. The arrangement is extremely irregular, giving the appearance of a complicated glomerulation — I call this site "the node*" (*k*). In the following sections, this bundle becomes gradually thicker and extends anteriorly. Consequently, the tip of the bundle protrudes into the fibrous septum (section No. 110). When projected to the left endocardial surface, the extension of the bundle occupies the posterior three quarters of the noncoronary aortic leaflet. The muscle fibers connect with the adjacent ordinary atrial muscle fibers (*v*) posteriorly and at the right hand margin of the node (Fig. 1 = section No. 110).

At the anterior border of the atrioventricular fibrous septum, and in the left subendocardial region, a muscle bundle (*l*) appears covered with thick connective tissue, sharply demarcated from the ventricular septal musculature (section No. 111). The tip of the muscle bundle coming from the atrial septum extends somewhat anteriorly to the left deeply into the connective tissue of the atrioventricular fibrous septum (*s*). In the next section, a muscle bundle (*h*) appears between the above-mentioned two muscle groups (Fig. 2 = section No. 112). The site is in the middle of the connective tissue of the lowest part of the membranous septum which separates the atrial musculature from the ventricular septal musculature.

In the next sections, the two posterior muscle groups (*k* and *h*) become longer and larger, breaking through the atrioventricular fibrous septum finally to combine together and make one muscle bundle (in section No. 114). The combined muscle bundle begins at the right anterior corner of the atrial septum and extends anteriorly in a gentle arch. The bundle is surrounded by thick connective tissue. On the left side, the bundle is separated from the left endocardium below the noncoronary and right coronary aortic leaflets. On the right side, it is separated from the ventricular septal muscle (*km*). The anterior tip of the bundle becomes longer and bigger, turning slightly to the right anteriorly and protruding

---

*Knoten

into a thick connective tissue mass which separates it from the ordinary ventricular musculature. The diameter of the stem (*h*) of the bundle is about 0.7 mm.

The most anterior muscle bundle (*l*) gradually lengthens posteriorly as well as anteriorly and always stays under the left endocardium. On the right side, it is separated from the ordinary septal musculature by thick connective tissue. The thick posterior tip finally connects with the stem of the bundle (*h*), not with the anterior tip of the stem but with its side at a definite angle (it was 60° in this specimen), forming a Y shape. The posterior stem (*h*) extends into the atrium, forming the atrioventricular node (*k*). The node is an irregularly arranged plexus of fibers. The thin left bundle branch (*l*) runs anteriorly, tapering gradually in the subendo-cardium, while the short thick right bundle branch (*r*) has a blunt tip. Both of the bundle branches (*l* and *r*) are completely separated from the ordinary ventricular musculature (*km*) by thick connective tissue (Fig. 3 = section No. 116).

In the subsequent sections, the connective tissue gradually thickens at the site of branching of the right bundle branch, finally separating the right bundle branch from the stem (in section No. 118). In the sections which follow, the separated right bundle branch, enclosed in thick connective tissue, extends further to the right anteriorly in the ventricular musculature. The left bundle branch (*l*) still forms the continuation of the stem (*h*). It extends anteriorly but not so rapidly as before. The length of the left bundle branch is almost equal to that of the stem, while the length of the right bundle branch here is approximately only half that of the stem (Fig. 4 = section No. 118).

In the following sections, at the point of penetration through the atrioventricular fibrous septum, much more connective tissue gradually appears, so that the stem (*h*) at this site gradually becomes more slender and is penetrated both lengthwise and crosswise by connective tissue so as to be divided into many small muscle islands and, finally, to be interrupted (section No. 122). Its anterior tip continues to the left bundle branch (*l*), so that it is difficult to draw a dividing line between them. On the other hand, the right bundle branch has already moved considerably toward the right anteriorly, and there exists a wide muscular zone of the ventricular septum (*km*) between the two bundle branches. The right bundle branch rapidly shortens and its cross-section becomes more and more oval. This means that the course of the right bundle branch rapidly turns inferiorly at this point. On the left side, it is separated from the adjacent ventricular septal musculature by a thin connective tissue sheath. On the right side, it is separated from the right ventricular cavity by a thick connective tissue sheath arising from a tendinous fiber (*sf*) for the septal leaflet of the tricuspid valve (Fig. 5 = section No. 125).

In the subsequent sections, the atrioventricular fibrous septum, joining the attachments of the mitral and tricuspid valves, becomes further thickened. The main stem (*h*) gradually becomes thinner until the posterior tip is completely replaced by connective tissue. The left bundle branch, several fibers thick, slowly moves anteriorly. The left bundle branch can be followed to the last section (No. 138) of this preparation. Throughout its course, it (*l*) lies in the subendocardium and is separated from the septal musculature by connective tissue on the right. The connective tissue is relatively thick everywhere except for a few sites (Fig. 6 = section No. 134).

The right bundle branch (*r*), becoming smaller and more round, gradually moves anteriorly. On its right side, the bundle branch is bordered by the connective tissue mass, which gradually becomes thinner. On its left, it is separated by a barely recognizable connective tissue layer from the adjacent ventricular musculature. I could follow the bundle branch only until section No. 135, because it was out of the preparation in the following sections. The right bundle branch became tiny in the last section, so that it was difficult to differentiate it from the surrounding ventricular musculature by weak magnification. The muscle fibers of neither of the bundle branches connected at any point with the ventricular musculature.

In the atrium, I recognized the peculiar muscle bundle (*k*) easily even after its separation from the stem (*h*) (after section No. 122). It attaches close to the right side of the atrioventricular fibrous septum in a broad manner, and lies close to the attachment of the septal leaflet of the tricuspid valve. The bundle is penetrated in many places by connective tissue originating from the atrioventricular fibrous septum (*s*). The size, however, gradually decreases inferiorly. In this case, even though it became small, I followed it up to section No. 134.

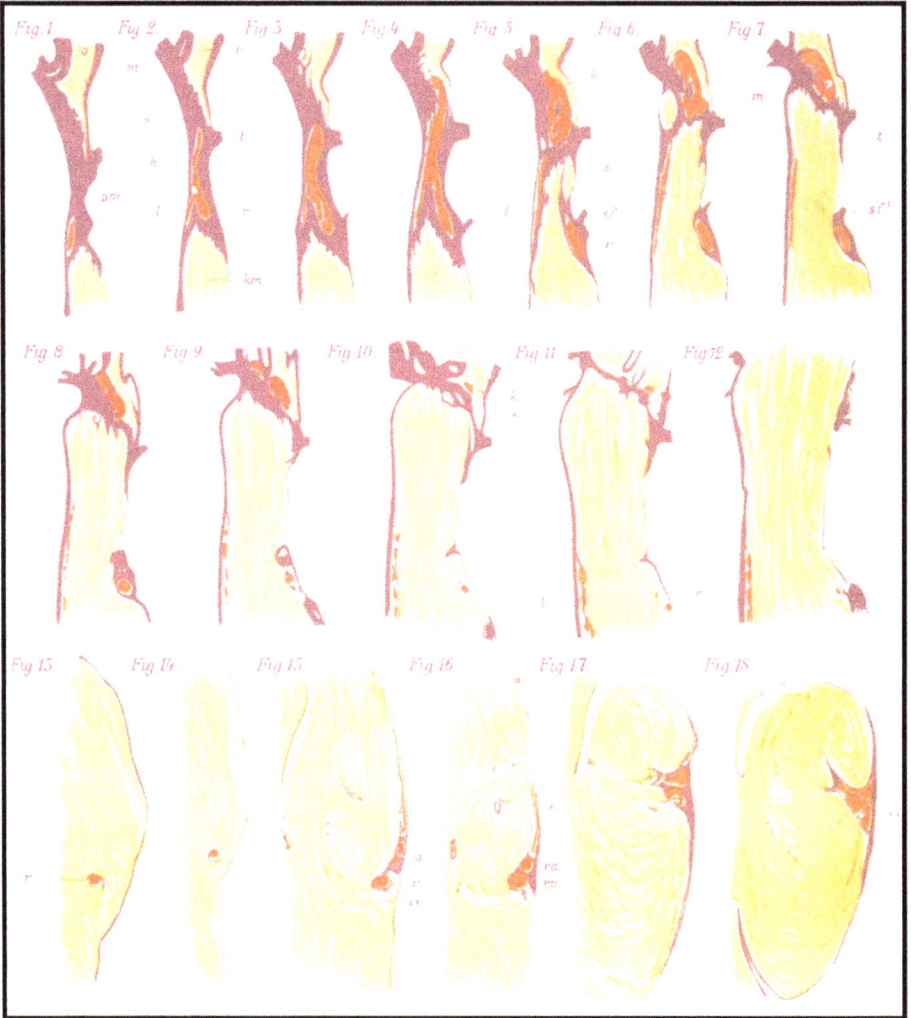

Human heart No. 143

v, *m*, *t*, *km*, *s*, *h*, *k*, *l*, *r* and *sf* are the same as for human heart No. 136.

pm = lowest portion of the membranous septum

After Fig. 13, magnification is higher than in Figs. 1–12; the figures contain only the right bundle branch

x, *ra* & *rp* (see text)

xx = a retrogradely running twig of the right bundle branch (cf. text)

A, *B*, *C*, *B'* and *xxx* = twigs of the right bundle branch

(*continued on next page*)

(continued from previous page)

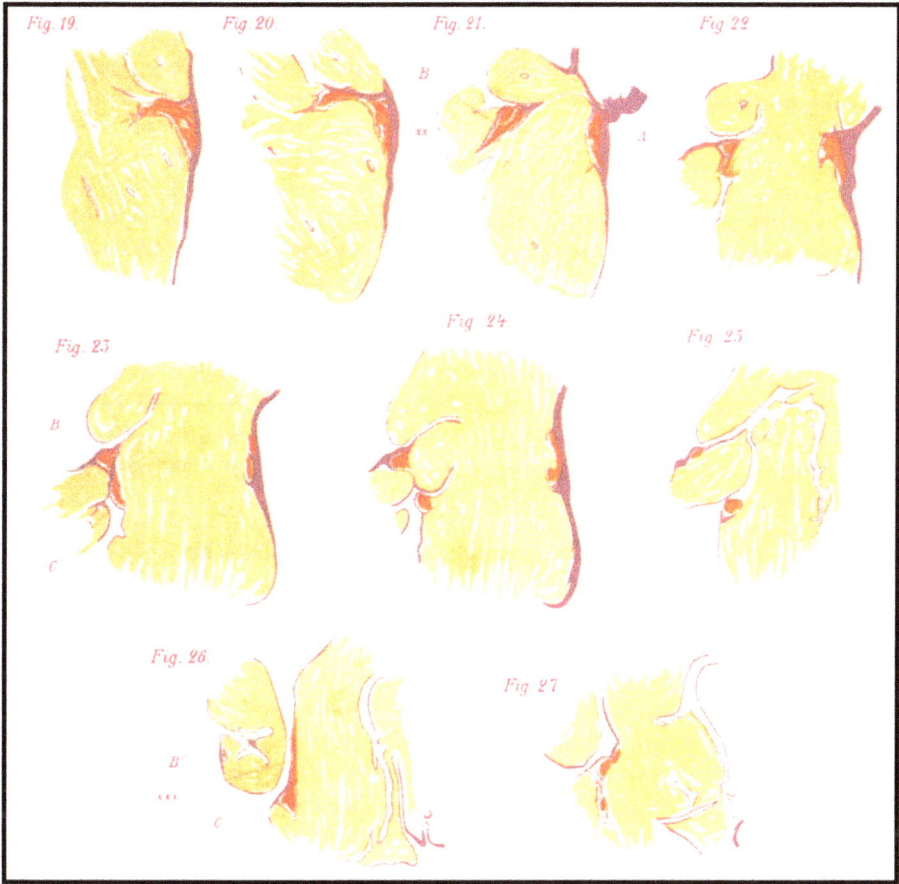

(2) *No. 143. The three-year-old child heart*

Preparation No. I was serially sectioned parallel to the free margin of the noncoronary aortic valvar leaflet, horizontally from the top to the bottom. The thickness of each section was 12 microns. Every fifth section was mounted and stained.

Through serial examination of the sections of preparation No. I, a special long, small muscle bundle is found for the first time at the level of the line connecting the lowest attachments of the noncoronary and right coronary leaflets of the aortic valve. It is located in the middle of this line, under the left endocardium of the ventricular septum and at the point corresponding to the anteroinferior margin of the membranous septum. The bundle is separated by a thick connective tissue mass from the ventricular septal musculature (Fig. 1 = section No. 2). In the next two sections, the bundle becomes somewhat larger and extends posteriorly. On the left side of this long, thin bundle appears a relatively thick process extending to the right and anteriorly so that the bundle forms a V shape (section No. 4).

In the following sections (sections No. 5–8), the posterior tip of the bundle enlarges significantly and extends posteriorly. The bundle is now Y-shaped. On the other hand, the right bundle branch (*r*) becomes thicker and advances somewhat anteriorly and to the right, ending with its blunt tip in a thick mass of connective tissue. The right bundle branch forms a leftward convex prominent stem with a posterior extension (*h*). The left bundle branch (*l*), therefore, looks just like a relatively thin appendage of the stem. So far, in the atrial septum, no special muscle bundle has been recognizable. The posteriorly extending stem has already reached behind the attachment of the septal leaflet of the tricuspid valve (*t*), but it is still separated by the thick atrioventricular fibrous septum (*s*) from the atrial musculature (*v*). The bifurcating anterior tip of the bundle sits astride the posterior edge of the ventricular musculature (*km*) with two legs (*r* and *l*). The two legs of the bundle are separated by a thick V-formed mass of connective tissue. Here, the anterior tips of both these legs extend anteriorly to the same extent (Fig. 2 = section No. 6).

In the following sections (sections No. 9–11), the posterior portion of the ventricular musculature gradually becomes sharper and longer, and protrudes further between the two branches of the Y-shaped muscle bundle.

The right bundle branch (*r*) also gradually extends anteriorly and to the right. Fibers, initially cut longitudinally in the posterior portion, are here cut more transversely. This fact indicates that the course of the right bundle branch is now directed inferiorly. The left bundle branch (*l*) extends somewhat anteriorly. The stem (*h*) also extends slightly posteriorly and widens. The stem always lies in the left subendocardium and also in the right subendocardium; the right endocardium, however, is much thicker. In this case, in section No. 11, there first appears in the atrium a half-moon-shaped special muscle mass which attaches to the atrioventricular fibrous septum. It is partly separated from the atrial musculature by connective tissue originating from the fibrous septum (Fig. 3 = section No. 10).

In the subsequent sections (No. 12–14), the stem of the Y-shaped bundle extending posteriorly now connects with the half-moon-shaped musculature (*k*). As far as both the bundle branches are concerned, there are no significant changes. The posterior portion of the right bundle branch, however, is divided into many areas by irregular netlike connective tissue which appeared earlier (Fig. 4 = section No. 14). Meanwhile, the connection between the atrial (*k*) and the ventricular (*h*) portion of the bundle becomes more extensive. The atrial portion lies on the right half of the septum. A significant change is now seen in the middle and the anterior portion of the connecting bundle. Connective tissue at the site of division of both the bundle branches (*l* and *r*) becomes thicker, especially around the right bundle branch. Consequently, the posterior portion of the right bundle branch finally becomes a group of muscular islands. The left bundle branch (*l*) is still connected with the stem (*h*). The mass of the stem decreases due to an increase of connective tissue and the left bundle branch seems to become relatively longer (sections No. 15–18).

In the following sections (No. 19–21), the ventricular septal musculature rapidly extends posteriorly and to the right, and reaches the site of attachment of the septal leaflet of the tricuspid valve (*t*). The left bundle branch is also divided into many groups of muscle fibers by connective tissue and finally becomes separated from the main stem (*h*) at its posterior tip. The posterior part of the right bundle branch gradually disappears and is recognizable only as several islands. The anterior tip of the right bundle branch, nonetheless, remains a longish oval as seen in cross section. Lying in the right subendocardium, the right bundle branch is embedded in a thick connective tissue mass, from the posterosuperior tip of which a tendinous fiber (*sf*) for the tricuspid valve originates. The main stem (*h*), which is penetrated liberally by coarse or fine connective tissue, can be seen only in its posterior part, which looks like isolated islands. The connective tissue between the main stem and the ventricular musculature continues (section No. 21) with the attachment of the tricuspid valve (*t*) on the right and that of the mitral valve (*m*) on the left, so that the atrioventricular fibrous septum again appears here. While the main stem disappears on the ventricular side, a considerable muscle bundle (*k*) can be seen on the atrial side (Fig. 5 = section No. 20).

In the subsequent sections (No. 22–30), the atrioventricular fibrous septum (*s*) gradually becomes thicker. The special muscle bundle can always be recognized in the atrium by its peculiar appearances, i.e. its irregularly interwoven netlike fiber arrangements, its special form of nuclei and its specific staining characteristics. Here, the muscle bundle lies as an irregular half-moon shape with the convex side to the right and somewhat posteriorly. It appears not to be sharply demarcated from the atrial musculature. On the other hand, the irregular and concave side of the bundle lies directly upon the fibrous septum. The bundle itself is penetrated multiply by connective tissue running in different directions, and part of the convex side is sharply bordered by connective tissue. It must be mentioned that the right anterior half of the bundle is separated by connective tissue, originating from the right part of the atrioventricular fibrous septum, from thin muscle fibers running subendocardially from the atrium to the base of the septal leaflet of the tricuspid valve. The characteristic muscle group (*k*) is the atrial segment of the connecting bundle. On the other hand, the subendocardial left bundle branch (*l*) continuously becomes thinner and loses its length, i.e. its horizontal width from posterior, while its anterior tip stays in an identical position. The left bundle branch is separated here by thin connective tissue from the ventricular septal musculature (*km*) which contacts directly with the atrioventricular fibrous septum posteriorly and occupies most of the thickness of the septal wall. The position of the right bundle branch (*r*) remains unchanged, not advancing anteriorly, whilst the size reduces slightly from behind. The form is a longish oval (length about 2 mm, width about 1.7 mm). The right bundle branch is always surrounded by a connective tissue sheath which gradually reduces in its amount. This connective tissue sheath originates from a tendinous fiber attaching to the septal leaflet of the tricuspid valve (Figs. 6 and 7 = sections No. 25 and No. 30).

In the following sections (No. 31–39), the atrioventricular fibrous septum, which formerly appeared irregular, runs straighter and eventually connects obliquely with the base of the septal leaflet of the tricuspid valve and with the base of the mitral valve, while thickening toward the mitral valve. The whole thickness of the septum is occupied by the ventricular musculature which supports directly the atrioventricular fibrous septum. The posterior portion of the connecting bundle is still seen in the atrium, although it gradually becomes smaller and is located more centrally, close to the atrioventricular fibrous septum. The bundle is irregularly penetrated by strands of connective tissue of varying thickness. The left bundle branch is still easily recognized as it is separated by connective tissue from the ventricular musculature. It is, however, already very thin and does not run as a bundle but is divided into many groups by strands of connective tissue, which penetrate between each of the muscle fibers or groups of muscle fibers. The right bundle branch rapidly thins from behind and, in cross section, becomes more rounded (in section No. 36, it is almost round, with a diameter of about 0.7 mm). The connective tissue mass bordering the right bundle branch on the right gradually becomes thinner, and in this connective tissue mass, isolated muscle fibers gradually appear which eventually replace the connective tissue mass (in section No. 39). The right bundle branch, therefore, is now surrounded by the ventricular musculature, and is separated from this musculature only by a very thin layer of connective tissue (Figs. 8 and 9 = sections No. 35 and No. 39).

In the subsequent sections (No. 40–48), a small remnant of the connecting bundle is still seen in the atrium. The right bundle branch is easily recognized by its form and location. Here, it is completely embedded within the ventricular musculature (in this case, approximately 0.5 mm away from the endocardium) and is covered by a connective tissue sheath. This sheath, however, is already very thin, and the thickness does not differ significantly from that of the interfascicular connective tissue of the adjacent septal musculature. The shape of the bundle branch as seen in these sections is initially round but it becomes more oval in lower sections (in section No. 48, the length is about 0.7 mm and the width about 0.4 mm; Fig. 10 = section No. 47).

In the following sections (sections No. 49–57), the remnant of the bundle is still seen in the atrium. The right bundle branch (*r*) is specifically recognized. Its size does not change, although its form and location change a little. The posterior part of the bundle branch gradually reduces in size and the anterior part enlarges. The right bundle branch consequently moves forward little by little as the number of the section progresses. The connective tissue covering the bundle branch appears not to decrease (Fig. 11 = section No. 56).

In the sections following No. 58, the right bundle branch, covered by a small amount of connective tissue, runs further inferiorly and somewhat anteriorly in the previously mentioned way. Here, the form and the size do not change. From section No. 60, the size again increases slightly, and the appearance becomes more and more similar to that of the surrounding ventricular musculature. Had I not examined the sections very carefully, I would almost be unable to differentiate the bundle branch from the ventricular musculature. In this way, I followed the right bundle branch up to section No. 79. Unfortunately, this section was the last to be used for detecting the right bundle branch of preparation No. I (Fig. 12 = section No. 69).

The left bundle branch was always visible from section No. 40. The horizontal subendocardial width is about 6 mm. In contrast, it is very thin, at most 0.3 mm. The bundle branch is separated from the ventricular musculature by connective tissue. There are abundant connective tissue fibers so that the bundle is interrupted by these fibers at certain sites, becoming divided into several muscle groups. In addition, there are some muscle fibers running independently, separated from the other muscle fibers by relatively thick connective tissue. In the subsequent sections, the anterior division* of the left bundle branch gradually diverges from the larger posterior division and takes an anteroinferior course. Simultaneously, the muscle fibers of the anterior division themselves converge to form a small bundle which runs subendocardially further anteroinferiorly along a relatively wide trabeculation. The larger posterior division runs further

---

Abteilung

downward with a wide extension, moving slightly forward and becoming, at the same time, gradually wider. From section No. 77, a portion of the bundle gradually diverges as an independent small bundle from the anterior part of the posterior division and moves anteroinferiorly. This preparation ended at section No. 90. As far as it was seen, the left bundle branch was always separated from the adjacent ventricular musculature by varying amounts of connective tissue. At several sites where connective tissue is sparse, however, two kinds of muscle, namely a muscle fiber of the bundle and a ventricular muscle fiber, lie relatively close to each other. As to the question whether the muscle fibers of the left bundle branch connect with the ventricular muscle fibers during their course up to here (up to 7 mm below the lowest attachment of the right coronary aortic leaflet), I must claim that they do not. I did not find these connections anywhere in this preparation, even after very careful examination.

From the findings described above, I was forced to pursue the further course of the right bundle branch in the remainder of the heart, which was still preserved in alcohol. I made, therefore, a new preparation which continued directly from the preparation described above (No. I). The new block was serially sectioned at 9-micron thickness and every 10th section was examined.

In this preparation, No. II, the continuation of the right bundle branch is readily visible. Here, the bundle lies about 0.8 mm away from the endocardium, surrounded by ventricular musculature but separated from it by thin fibers of connective tissue as well as rather wide lymphatics. The shape is round (the diameter here is about 0.3 mm) and fine connective tissue can clearly be seen between the muscle fibers of the bundle (Fig. 13 = section No. 6-II). No such fine connective tissue is seen between the adjacent ordinary ventricular muscle fibers.

In the sections which follow, the right bundle branch shows no changes in terms of its position, size and shape. The fibers are sectioned transversely, indicating that the bundle here takes an almost vertical course downward. As the sections progress, the shape of the bundle gradually becomes irregular, changing into a triangle with an obtuse angle in sections No. 13–20. Hereafter, the bundle gradually becomes a longish oval and, at the same time, somewhat smaller. (In section No. 33, the longer diameter is about 0.4 mm and the shorter diameter is about 0.2 mm.) The fibers of connective tissue between each muscle fiber gradually diminish and, instead, several rather wide lymphatics appear between the muscle fibers, dividing them into two or three groups.

In the subsequent sections, the cross-sectional shape of the bundle branch gradually becomes smaller and round again, with the form being almost circular in section No. 43 (the diameter is about 0.25 mm). Hereafter, the size again increases little by little and the diameter is about 0.5 mm in section No. 59. In this preparation, after section No. 4, the bundle gradually approaches the endocardium so that the distance from the endocardial surface is about 0.25 mm in section No. 60. There is, however, a very thin layer of ventricular septal muscle between the bundle and the endocardium. During its long course up to here, there are neither direct connections nor contacts between the bundle and the ventricular musculature. The bundle is always separated from the ventricular musculature by connective tissue fibers of varying thickness and, in some sites, by relatively wide lymphatics (Fig. 14 = section No. 45-II).

From here, the right bundle branch shows a conspicuous change. In section No. 60, the bundle is no longer surrounded by the ventricular musculature on all its sides. The anterior boundary is formed by a very thick and strong mass of connective tissue in the subendocardium. In this connective tissue, three or four round small muscle bundles appear which lie separately in a line and are also completely separated from the connecting bundle by thick connective tissue (Fig. 15 = section No. 60-II).

In the next sections, the newly appeared muscle bundles enlarge very rapidly and the mass of connective tissue separating them also rapidly decreases. Consequently, the bundles are gathered into a muscle group and are surrounded by a common connective tissue sheath. At the time when the muscle bundles appear, part of the connecting bundle, which still has a round cross-section and is divided into many muscle bundles by fine connective tissue fibers and lymphatics, spreads forward. This part of the connecting bundle gradually joins the newly appeared muscle bundles (section No. 56). Thereafter, this bundle is again divided into two groups by connective tissue. The posterior muscle group (*rp*), consisting exclusively of the muscle fibers of the connecting bundle, maintains a round shape. On the other hand, the anterior muscle group (*ra*), consisting of the newly appeared muscle mass and part of the bundle just separated from the connecting bundle, has an oval shape. The anterior group rapidly becomes bigger and is divided into several areas by numerous wide lymph gaps and thin connective tissue. From its anterior tip, a very small process having several muscle fibers (Fig. 16, *x*) extends anteriorly in the subendocardium. This process runs rather a long distance in the subendocardium and finally connects with the ordinary ventricular musculature. The two muscle groups lie close to each other beneath the endocardium. They are separated from the ventricular musculature by thick connective tissue posteriorly and anteriorly on the left (sections No. 61–67; Fig. 16 = section No. 65-II).

In the sections which follow (No. 68–80), the size and form of the posterior muscle group (*rp*) gradually becomes smaller and more irregular. On the other hand, the anterior muscle group (*ra*) enlarges gradually, whilst the anterior tip shortens. In section No. 74-II, the anterior group is much larger than the posterior, and the connective tissue fibers separating the two muscle groups become scarcer and finally disappear. These two muscle groups then join together into one muscle group (section No. 75), with the form of a scalene quadrangle (Figs. 17 and 18 = sections No. 72 and No. 78-II). This muscle bundle is also divided into many muscle bundles by wide lymphatics and delicate connective tissue fibers, especially at the thinner left half. This portion is separated from the ventricular musculature on three sides by an especially thick mass of connective tissue. Each of the muscle fibers or muscle groups of the bundle are scattered like islands. The right bundle branch gradually becomes very big after section No. 45, as shown in the figures.

Here, I would like to mention one thing. A small muscle bundle (Figs. 16–18, *xx*), not belonging to the connecting bundle but to the ventricular musculature and lying outside the connective tissue sheath of the bundle, gradually penetrates into the sheath (section No. 68). Moreover, this small muscle bundle, always surrounded by a connective tissue sheath, advances between the muscle fibers of the connecting bundle and subsequently courses inferiorly surrounded on all sides by the muscle fibers of the connecting bundle (section No. 75).

The preparation (No. II) ended again with section No. 80. The right bundle branch, however, does not end but rather seems gradually to enlarge again. I, therefore, made yet another preparation, which is the direct inferior continuation of preparation No. II and which contains the right bundle branch. In this preparation No. III, I did not utilize the full thickness but, as in preparation No. II, only used the right half of the septum, where the right bundle branch is presumed to exist. The preparation included numerous trabeculations extending either to the base of the anterior papillary muscle or to the parietal wall.

In preparation No. III, the right bundle branch is again recognized very easily. Here, however, the muscle fibers of the right bundle branch are no longer cut transversely but longitudinally. The form of the bundle is still an irregular quadrangle. One side, lying in the subendocardium, is rather long (1.5 mm), and the opposite side is much shorter (about 0.4 mm). The other two sides (the anterior and the posterior) are relatively long (about 1.6 mm), forming an arch toward the inside of the quadrangle (Fig. 19 = section No. 3-III). In the following sections, the posterior side arches much more inwardly, so that the quadrangle is constricted at the middle and is consequently separated into two portions (Fig. 20 = section No. 10-III).

So far, the bundle has always coursed along a trabeculation. Now, after dividing into two bundles, one bundle (*A*) runs continuously along the trabeculation, but the other bundle (*B*) goes into another trabeculation. The first bundle (*A*) contains more connective tissue between the muscle fiber groups than the adjacent ventricular musculature does. This bundle is separated from the ventricular musculature by more or less prominent connective tissue fibers and partly by wide lymphatic spaces. The bundle gradually becomes thinner, but the area of subendocardial extension seems to increase. However, it disappears finally in section No. 30-III (Figs. 21–24).

The ventricular muscle bundle (*xx*), which invaded between the muscle groups of the connecting bundle as stated above in section No. 68 of preparation No. II, runs inferiorly together with the connecting bundle and remains within the connective tissue sheath of the bundle (*A*). It is separated from the connecting bundle by a particularly fine connective tissue sheath together with wide lymphatic spaces, and gradually becomes smaller. The border of the ventricular muscle bundle, after losing its own connective tissue sheath and approaching much closer to the muscle fibers of the connecting bundle, becomes indistinct (in section No. 20-III). At the beginning, this small ventricular muscle bundle has all the characteristics of ventricular musculature and is easily differentiated from the connecting bundle by its dark tincture, abundant nuclei and smaller fibers. As it courses downward, however, these characteristics gradually change and approximate to those of the connecting bundle, so that finally (in section No. 20) no definite differentiation can be made.

The other twig (*B*) of the right bundle branch is triangular, and one side lies in the subendocardium. In the following sections, the tip opposite to the subendocardium becomes elongated. The elongated portion (*C*) is finally separated from the other half (*B*) by connective tissue which gradually becomes thicker (section No. 20). The separated portion (*C*) moves to another trabeculation, again lying in the subendocardium. The bundle (*B*) encloses a special ventricular muscle in its middle. This ventricular muscle originating from the adjacent ventricular musculature had previously entered the right bundle branch before it divided (in sections No. 2–6-III). The muscle, surrounded by connective tissue fibers and lymphatic spaces, ran downward with the connecting bundle. This enclosed ventricular muscle gradually enlarges and connects again with the adjacent ventricular musculature (sections No. 32–34-III). It appears that the ventricular muscle does not connect directly with the muscle fibers of the bundle (*B*), as could be presumed. The small bundle (*B*) goes further inferiorly separated from the ventricular musculature by wide lymphatic spaces, and is finally divided into two finer muscle groups (in section No. 43 = Fig. 26). I could not follow these fine twigs up to their terminations.

The third bundle (*C*) runs inferiorly with a round cross-section (about 0.5 mm in diameter), separated from the ventricular musculature by connective tissue fibers and lymphatic spaces. During its course, the bundle becomes slightly bigger and gradually longer until a long process of muscle fibers stretches from the bundle in the subendocardium (Fig. 26, *xxx*). The main mass becomes smaller in the following sections, and is again divided into two groups. The smaller one becomes separated from the other and presumably moves into another trabeculation. In contrast, the bigger one continues to run its original course and again is divided into two groups by connective tissue (section No. 55). I could not pursue all of these fine terminal twigs any more, because this preparation (No. III) unfortunately ended at this point. The position is about 23 mm away from the inferior margin of the membranous interventricular septum. Here, the endocardium of the muscular ventricular septum continues anteriorly to join that of the right ventricular parietal wall, in other words, the anterior corner of the ventricular septum. At this corner, there are trabeculations of various sizes running in various directions and either ramifying, crossing each other, or bridging the transitional zone from the septum to the parietal wall. The terminal twigs of the right bundle branch here proceed to the right ventricular parietal wall through several trabeculations. In particular, the bundle (*B*) reaches the anterior papillary muscle through one of these trabeculations and spreads at the base of the papillary muscle into many fine twigs (Figs. 21–27 = sections No. 14, 18, 24, 28, 34, 43 and 51-III).

(3) *No. 139. The heart of a female fetus, 31.5 cm long*

The lower part of the ventricles, including the apex, was cut away from this fetal heart. The upper larger part of the ventricles, together with the atrial chambers and the original portion of the great arterial trunks, was fixed in alcohol, embedded in paraffin and serially sectioned in 9-micron thickness posteroanteriorly, parallel to the long axis of the heart and vertical to the septum. Every sixth section was retained and stained first with Haematoxylin and then with van Gieson.

In section No. 8, a peculiar muscle bundle (*k*) appears in the atrial septum (*v*) close to the atrioventricular fibrous septum (*s*). On the left side, the fibrous septum originates broadly from the base of the mitral valve (*m*) and extends rightward and inferiorly toward the base of the septal leaflet of the tricuspid valve (*t*), with a slight curve and a gradual decrease in size. The half-moon-shaped bundle attaches with its concave surface to the fibrous septum. Here, it is not distinctly separated from the adjacent atrial musculature. Instead, there are connections between them. In contrast, it is distinctly separated from the ventricular musculature by the thick connective tissue of the atrioventricular septum (*s*) (Fig. 1 = section No. 9).

In the following sections, the bundle (*k*) gradually becomes bigger and can be differentiated more easily from the atrial musculature, while being bordered on its left and superiorly by thin connective tissue originating from the left end of the fibrous septum. It should be noted that the directions of the muscle fibers of the bundle are quite different from those of the adjacent atrial musculature. The fibers of the bundle are sectioned

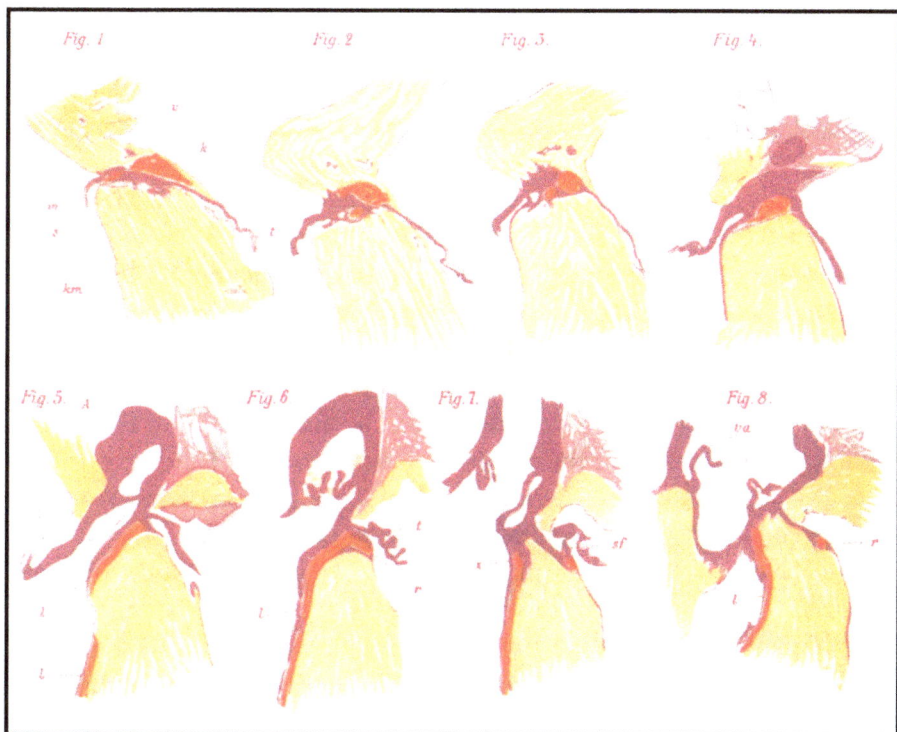

Human heart No. 139

- v = the atrial septum
- k = node, i.e. atrial segment of the connecting system
- m = the anterior mitral leaflet
- t = septal leaflet of the tricuspid valve
- s = the atrioventricular fibrous septum
- km = ventricular septum
- l & r = the left and the right bundle branch of the connecting system
- sf = a tendinous fiber for septal leaflet of the tricuspid valve
- l' & x (see text)
- va = leaflets of the aortic valve

almost transversely, whilst those of the atrial musculature are mostly sectioned longitudinally. This makes it easy to differentiate the two components at a glance. Abundant connective tissue from the fibrous septum is projected into the peculiar muscle bundle, not so much at the beginning, but gradually many projections penetrate the muscle bundle in various directions. The atrioventricular fibrous septum gradually increases in breadth, forming an irregular network. Accordingly, the gaps of the network are filled completely with the peculiar muscle masses (section No. 14).

In the sections which follow, the peculiar muscle groups proceed more and more toward the ventricular side of the atrioventricular septum and, in section No. 18, the muscle can be seen beyond the fibrous septum, being separated from the ventricular musculature by fine connective tissue. The main mass of the bundle still remains on the atrial side, increasing its size gradually and taking its site at the right inferior portion of the most anterior part of the atrial septum (Fig. 2 = section No. 19).

After section No. 20, the muscle bundle (k), which is still visible on the atrial side, becomes somewhat smaller and round. It is bordered by thick connective tissue of the fibrous septum on the left and the right, and is separated by relatively thick connective tissue from the ventricular musculature inferiorly. Superiorly, there are still connections with the ordinary atrial musculature. In section No. 23, for the first time, the bundle is surrounded by connective tissue on all sides. In this section, it lies completely within the fibrous septum, also being separated from the atrium by a thin layer of connective tissue. It is irregularly penetrated by connective tissue of variable thickness originating from the fibrous septum. The diameter of the muscle bundle is here about 0.9 mm (Fig. 3 = section No. 23).

In the following sections (No. 24–29), the connective tissue between the bundle and the atrial musculature becomes gradually thicker and joins the atrioventricular fibrous septum. The bundle gradually takes an oval shape and lies just below the fibrous septum and above the ventricular septal musculature. It is separated from the ventricular musculature on the right by a minimal layer of connective tissue, and on the left by a somewhat wider layer of connective tissue. The left half of the bundle, which here is still oval, is penetrated by rather thick connective tissue and is divided into several fields. Most of the muscle fibers of the bundle are here sectioned transversely.

In the next sections (sections No. 30–35), the oval form changes slowly. The left tip lengthens inferiorly in the subendocardium. The muscle fibers, and the connective tissue within, also lead in the same direction. The muscle fibers in the right half seem mostly directed anteriorly. In section No. 35, the bundle shows the following configuration. It begins with a thick round head close to the base of the septal leaflet of the tricuspid valve. It lies beneath the lowest attachment of the noncoronary leaflet of the aortic valve and stretches obliquely to the left and inferiorly like a tail up to the thick subendocardial connective tissue on the left side (Fig. 4 = section No. 30).

From section No. 36, the connecting bundle lengthens more and more to the left and inferiorly (*l*). In section No. 36, in its lowest part, two peculiar muscle bundles appear in the subendocardium on the left, which are separated from each other by connective tissue. The histological features are similar to those of the bundle higher in the subendocardium, although there is no connection between them. They are also separated from the ventricular musculature by connective tissue. In the sections which follow, the two lower bundles gradually join together into one bundle (*l'*) and lengthen superiorly (Fig. 5 = section No. 39).

In section No. 40, at the right end of the connecting bundle which up to now has remained unchanged, a small process directed to the right and inferiorly can be identified. In the subsequent sections, the process (*r*) gradually becomes elongated (sections No. 41–45). The left bundle branch extends more and more inferiorly but becomes thinner at the same time. Eventually, the left bundle branch connects with the endocardial muscle bundle mentioned above (*l'*), which has extended from inferiorly to superiroly. The whole connecting bundle, therefore, forms a very thin half moon shape, enveloping the top of the ventricular septal musculature with its concave side from up and left like an arch. The bundle and the ventricular musculature are always more or less sharply separated from each other by layers of connective tissue. In particular, the connective tissue mass at the top of the ventricular muscle is thick (Fig. 6 = section No. 46).

In section No. 47, the root of the right bundle branch is narrowed both above and below by connective tissue, and is subsequently separated from the left bundle branch in the sections which follow. The distance between the two bundle branches rapidly becomes greater while the connective tissue mass, covering the top of the ventricular musculature in a reversed V shape, thrusts upward indenting the right and the left bundle branch from the lower medial side. This connective tissue mass is already joined to the fibrous septum by the tip of the inverted V figure (in section No. 47). The combination becomes tighter, and now forms an inverted Y in section No. 50, separating the two bundle branches from the ventricular musculature.

The left bundle branch (*l*) has already extended here a long distance inferiorly in the form of a thin striation. On the left side, the bundle branch is bordered by rather thick subendocardial connective tissue, on the right upper side by the Y-shaped connective tissue mass just mentioned, and on the right lower side it is separated by quite thin connective tissue from the ventricular musculature. The upper portion of the bundle branch is thicker (about 0.5 mm thick) but it becomes gradually thinner inferiorly. At the lowest portion, I could no longer differentiate it with certainty from the ventricular musculature. This is because connective tissue fibers separating the two muscle groups are too sparse to differentiate them, and the bundle here is too loose due to penetrating connective tissue.

After separating from the left bundle branch, the left upper end of the right bundle branch shortens rapidly. The right bundle branch, however, gradually lengthens toward the right and somewhat inferiorly. In section No. 50, it takes an egg shape, directing its broader pole toward the right and inferiorly and its narrower pole toward the left and superiorly. Inferiorly on the left, it is separated from the ventricular musculature by one of the legs of the Y-shaped connective tissue mass, and superiorly on the right it is bordered by a layer of thick subendocardial connective tissue (sections No. 47–50).

In the following sections (No. 51–55), the ventricular musculature extends further upward and directly meets with the fibrous septum. Two legs of the Y-shaped connective tissue surrounding the ventricular musculature become separated from each other and eventually lose their common stem. The legs persist on both the right and left sides as completely separated processes of connective tissue (Fig. 7, *x*). The left bundle branch (*l*) does not change much except that the upper portion shortens. The right bundle branch (*r*) becomes gradually smaller and moves slightly downward. It is still surrounded by a thick connective tissue mass on all sides. In section No. 53, a tendinous fiber (*sf*) for the septal leaflet of the tricuspid valve arises from this connective tissue (Fig. 7 = section No. 53).

From section No. 56, the left bundle branch (*l*) gradually becomes thinner and the direction of the individual muscle fibers is somewhat different from that of the neighboring ventricular musculature (*km*). The two kinds of muscle (*l* and *km*) are always separated from each other by connective tissue. The connective tissue fibers, however, become so scarce inferiorly that I was almost unable to differentiate the two muscle groups with certainty. In section No. 63, I was finally unable to trace the left bundle branch because of the inappropriate direction of the sections. As can be easily seen from a simple cross-section of the total ventricle, the ventricular septum takes a concave curve toward the right. Because of this, it is impossible to produce exactly vertical serial sections of the septum from its posterior to its anterior end with geometrical accuracy.

The right bundle branch (*r*) gradually becomes smaller and moves further anteriorly and slightly downward (Fig. 8 = section No. 59). It has an oval cross-section and is surrounded by thick connective tissue on the upper left and on the right whilst its tip, directed to the right and downward, is separated by thin connective tissue from the ventricular musculature. The connective tissue combines with the fibrous septum, but this connection becomes attenuated until it finally disappears (in section No. 62). This connective tissue accompanying the right bundle branch becomes thinner and thinner, but it still remains as a considerable mass between the right bundle branch and the endocardium. A tendinous fiber* (in section No. 72) starts from the connective tissue where the bundle branch lies approximately 0.3 mm away from the right endocardium. Separated by a thin connective tissue sheath, the bundle branch is surrounded by the ventricular musculature on three sides (right, below and left). The lymph spaces of the connecting bundle at this point appear wider than those of the adjacent ventricular musculature. The right bundle branch does not become smaller hereafter but, on the contrary, seems to become gradually bigger and looser at the same time. The relatively thick connective tissue at the upper end gradually disappears (in section No. 78), and in this way the right bundle branch becomes surrounded on all sides by the ordinary muscle of the

---

*Sehnenfaden

ventricular septum, at the same time moving slowly inferiorly. From the microscopic appearance, it is hardly possible to differentiate the right bundle branch from the surrounding ordinary muscle fibers. When the serial sections are very carefully followed, however, it can be traced more inferiorly with certainty. In section No. 81, its shape is round (the diameter is about 0.16 mm). In section No. 84, it is divided into several small groups by lymph spaces, and having gradually elongated inferiorly (section No. 88), it becomes separated from the neighboring ventricular musculature by widening lymph spaces.

In the subsequent section, the right bundle branch changes its position rapidly downward. In section No. 96, it forms a long narrow spindle which is divided into many fiber groups by lymph spaces. After section No. 97, it lengthens very rapidly inferiorly and, in section No. 101, I could observe only its upper portion, because, to my regret, the lower half of the ventricle was cut away, as I previously mentioned. In the last few sections, the fibers were cut longitudinally. In other words, the fibers ran vertically from above down, the direction being the same as that of the adjacent ventricular muscle fibers.

In the entire course of the right bundle branch up to now, I could not confirm any connection between the bundle branch and the ordinary ventricular muscle fibers.

A further brief summary: the left bundle branch initially runs inferiorly as a broad and compact bundle, but diverges lower down and is separated from the ventricular musculature by connective tissue of varying thickness. In these serial preparations, I could not determine the most inferior extent of the left bundle branch, because the lower half of the ventricle was cut away. Anyway, it is certain that the bundle branch did not end before the middle of the left ventricle. This fact is contradictory to the statements of all other previous investigators. The question whether the muscle fibers of the left bundle branch connect anywhere in its course with the ordinary ventricular muscle fibers cannot be answered with certainty. The reason for this is that the preparation was badly stained, probably due to many years of preservation in alcohol. The presence of abundant connections between these two kinds of muscle, nonetheless, must surely be denied.

(4) *Macroscopic observation of the connecting bundle of the human heart*

I earlier described microscopic findings of part of the connecting bundle in the human heart. These were concerned, however, only with the atrial segment, the part of the connecting bundle between the atrium and the ventricle, and portions of the two bundle branches, i.e. the course of the right bundle branch up to the base of the anterior papillary muscle, and the uppermost course of the left bundle branch. As described previously, in all hearts the connecting bundle extends in the same way, taking the same position and the same form in the area stated above. The right bundle branch is always smaller than the left bundle branch, and is separated from the ventricular musculature by a more or less thick layer of connective tissue. The left bundle branch is wide where it begins, and it becomes wider and at the same time thinner as it extends downward, consequently splitting into many groups. I could not microscopically pursue their extension further, because all of my preparations ended in this area.

Because I had not yet followed the left bundle branch up to its ending, I wanted to confirm microscopically the lower terminal, and I considered this goal not difficult to achieve. In spite of my efforts, however, I encountered great difficulties in continuing the study. After a long, vain endeavor, I was forced to interrupt the study.

I first tried to determine how far downward the left bundle branch extends. This apparently simple question was very difficult to answer. To investigate the extension of the left bundle branch, I cut from many hearts long vertical specimens from the lower margin of the membraneous septum to the cardiac apex. The long specimen, of several millimeters in width and thickness, was then divided into two or three pieces, because the whole piece was too long to be studied. These pieces were embedded and cut lengthwise. I assumed that, if the pieces were examined in an orderly way, it would be easy to find out where the extension of the left bundle branch terminated, and how the muscle bundle eventually connected with the ordinary ventricular musculature. In this way, I hoped to achieve my goal.

When the specimen was systematically examined, the subendocardial muscle fibers of the left bundle branch were always detected in the upper half of the specimen. When this muscle bundle was followed inferiorly, however, I encountered an inexplicable situation. The situation was as follows. The left bundle branch, surrounded by connective tissue, did not extend lower to the same distance in all of the hearts, but the extension varied significantly from heart to heart. Moreover, there were other unexpected findings. When examined further inferiorly, subendocardial muscle groups were seen scattering here and there. These muscle groups existed as a broad bundle, or as a small bundle with only a few fibers, being separated from the adjacent myocardium by a more or less thick layer of connective tissue. The subendocardial muscle groups were recognized in all of the hearts, but their number, size and position varied significantly among the hearts. When examined more precisely, the fiber directions of the muscle groups were seen to be varied, being crosswise, or oblique, or lengthwise. In the case first described, the individual muscle fibers were usually seen to run completely surrounded by subendocardial connective tissue. Because the directions of the muscle groups were generally quite different from those of the adjacent ventricular musculature, it was noted that there existed two different kinds of muscle group. It was sometimes found, nonetheless, that the two muscle groups extended in almost the same direction, and that there were not enough connective tissues separating the two muscle groups; in such cases, because the histological differences were not significant, if indeed any existed, it was not always easy to differentiate the two muscle groups.

From the findings described above, I was unable to clarify the architecture of the left bundle branch. I could not confirm the claims of all the previous investigators who insisted that the connecting bundle connected with the ventricular musculature soon after reaching the ventricular septum. I also could not answer the question whether the scattered muscle groups in the subendocardium in the lower half of the specimen were related to the left bundle branch in the upper half of the specimen. Further, I could not determine what kind of relationship existed between the two muscle groups. In spite of the ambiguity, however, I did not shrink from the very difficult task. I continued to undertake similar studies. I made sections by cutting in different directions; such as from the lower margin of the membranous septum, where the left bundle branch presumably originated, to the anteroinferior or to the posteroinferior. In the sections extending from the membranous septum to the posteroinferior direction, I was convinced that the left bundle branch did not extend far to the posterior. Its anterior and inferior margins, nonetheless, still remained unclear. I was eventually forced to give up this study.

In the meantime, I studied the hearts from cats and dogs. I also found in them the subendocardially scattered characteristic muscle bundles, but I could not find any relationship between these muscle bundles and the connecting bundle. During the study, the idea came to my mind that the peculiar muscle fibers might be the so-called Purkinje fibers. This idea became more and more convincing as I examined in more detail the hearts of cats, dogs and humans. This was because I always found the scattered subendocardial muscle groups in the ventricles of all the hearts examined, although there were some histological variations among them. Consequently, as suggested by Professor L. Aschoff, I examined the heart of a sheep (No. 155) in order to clarify the relationship between the subendocardial muscle groups and Purkinje fibers. This is because Purkinje fibers can be seen most clearly in the sheep heart. The result of the experiment was most surprising. With this first sheep heart, I was able completely to solve the riddle. I will present an exact description of the sheep heart later in a special chapter. Briefly, however, the atrioventricular bundle does not connect directly with the ventricular musculature as was believed before, but divides into two bundle branches and then spreads, as an independent system, further throughout the inner surfaces of both the ventricles as Purkinje fibers.

This discovery definitely facilitated my study, because I could then orientate the entire course of the connecting bundle far better than before. I then examined the heart of a calf, and renewed my study of the human, dog and cat hearts. I found an amazing constancy in the courses of the connecting bundle, except for a few small differences among animal species.

I made serial sections of the whole left ventricles of the sheep, dog and cat hearts, and described precisely the course of the left bundle branch. I did not use this method for the human heart, for the following reasons. First, the method is very difficult and time-consuming, and good results might not be expected in spite of such efforts because, in the human heart, there are strong histological similarities between the ordinary cardiac muscle fibers and those of the connecting bundle. Second, the left bundle branch was highly recognizable, even macroscopically, in almost all the human hearts, either in fresh or fixed condition. On the whole, the left bundle branch follows a definite, more or less uniform course, except for minor individual differences. In the following section I will present the macroscopic findings relating to the left bundle branch of the human heart. For macroscopic examination of the course of the left bundle branch, the fresh hearts and the hearts fixed with Kaiserling and kept in glycerin were almost equally useful, and most of the hearts fixed by other methods were also useful.

Macroscopic Observations of the Left Bundle Branch[*]

When the left ventricle is observed macroscopically in many hearts, it can be seen that the inner surfaces of various hearts are differently constructed to a greater or lesser extent. A uniform description, therefore, might not be appropriate. In general, however, the inner surfaces of the left ventricles of all hearts are similarly constructed. Without exception, the ventricular septal surface beneath the noncoronary leaflet of the aortic valve is relatively smooth, whereas the other part of the septum, together with the entire parietal wall, shows a great unevenness because of the presence of trabeculations everywhere except for the papillary muscles. The extent of the smooth portion differs greatly, though usually it is broadest in the vicinity of the aortic valve. It gradually becomes narrower as it extends downward, and it is connected with the area where many trabecular elevations and intertrabecular recesses are found. In dilated hearts, the smooth portion usually is extensive. The posterior papillary muscle usually consists not of one conical muscle mass, but of two or more muscle groups. They are usually fused interdependently, but not infrequently they are independent of each other. On the other hand, the anterior papillary muscle is composed usually of one muscle mass. The size of the trabeculations in the other parts of the wall varies considerably from heart to heart. In the ventricular septum, the trabeculations usually

---

[*]Photographs of the bundles of two human hearts together with tracings on which the course of the connecting bundle is drawn in red are given in Plate I, Figs. 1 and 2.

extend obliquely from anterosuperior to posteroinferior. Inferiorly, they are divided into many smaller trabeculations, which are fused with each other. At the lower third of the septum, especially between the two papillary muscles, the trabeculations usually form a reticular net. Individual trabeculations are generally round, but are relatively flat in some cases.

When the left ventricular endocardium is observed carefully, one finds in most cases that the endocardium is slightly thickened and unevenly opaque at the place directly beneath the right coronary leaflet of the aortic valve and the membranous septum, although no special structure is recognizable in the endocardium. When the endocardium is observed in this inferior area, an indistinctly striped configuration gradually appears in the opaque endocardium. These stripes extend either in separate groups from the outset, or extend diffusely at the beginning, converging into groups a little lower down. The direction of the stripes differs according to the height of the septum. In general, the stripes run downward in a diverging fashion, so they or their groups at the anterior zone of the smooth portion diverge more anteroinferiorly, while those at the posterior zone diverge more vertically downward or sometimes posteriorly, and those between the zones diverge inferiorly. The smooth opaque endocardium gradually becomes thinner and transparent in the inferior, anterior and posterior areas. The endocardium finally becomes a trabecular sheath. Meanwhile, the trabeculations, as well as the intertrabecular recesses, gradually become apparent through the endocardium. As the endocardium becomes more transparent, the stripes become more distinct. In other words, the stripes become much more apparent toward the inferior and the anterior areas. At the peripheral portion of the smooth endocardium, the stripes usually divide into groups as broad cords, but sometimes as narrow cords. They extend either subendocardially along the trabeculations or as free tendinous fiber-like cords through the ventricular cavity, or extend on the ventricular surface, making an endocardial fold. The stripes extend in various directions, mostly toward both the papillary muscles. The stripes running anteroinferiorly can usually be seen clearly, because they generally run crosswise to the underlying cardiac musculature. This description, nonetheless, concerns only the main stem of the left bundle branch.

The extent to which the left bundle branch is visible macroscopically differs greatly from specimen to specimen. In some hearts, it was very difficult to differentiate the main stem from the other mural structures. In other hearts, the left bundle branch was so clearly distinguishable that the course of every small bundle could be followed. One of the hearts in which the courses of even small bundles could easily be followed was a heart which was markedly dilated and hypertrophied due to mitral regurgitation, and which had been fixed in Formol-Müller solution and preserved in alcohol. In this heart, the trabeculations were mostly flattened, and the smooth portion of the endocardium was very extensive. In this smooth portion, and approximately 1 cm below the right coronary leaflet of the aortic valve, a vertically striped layer of fibers 1.2 cm wide diverged gradually downward. The anterior muscle fibers of the layer gradually separated from the other fibers and extended anteroinferiorly. The muscle fibers then converged to form a small bundle, entered a small (about 1 cm long) tendinous fiber-like cord, extended obliquely anteroinferiorly, attached to a trabeculation, and extended from there to the anterior papillary muscle. Like the fibers mentioned above, the other fibers, joining together to make numerous small muscle bundles no thicker than horsehairs, were also highly visible. They were arranged as a thin broad layer, took a downward course, and gradually divided into two divisions (a and p).

The posterior division (p) extended posteroinferiorly, and gradually divided again into many groups. Some small muscle bundles of this group converged posteroinferiorly, entered a tendinous fiber-like cord, and reached directly the middle portion of the posterior papillary muscle. The other muscle fibers of the posterior division advanced along their course, often combining with, as well as dividing from, each other. Some of the muscle fibers eventually extended to the posterior wall, some extended to the trabeculations of the base of the posterior papillary muscle, and others extended to the trabecular nets at the apex of the heart.

The anterior division (a) of small muscle bundles, as a whole, extended further inferiorly. The small bundles in this group were well recognized individually as fine gray fibers beneath the endocardium. They did not extend parallely in a downward direction, but combined with each other, divided into many finer fibers, or crossed each other. As a consequence, they formed many long, narrow nets. In general, the long axis of the nets was vertical. The small muscle bundles of the anterior division reached the anteroinferior border of the smooth endocardium and converged gradually into three groups, each of which entered one of three short cords. The cords joined together, entered a thin and broad membrane covered by the endocardium on both sides, and attached to a trabeculation. Further from this trabeculation, the cords ran to the base of the anterior papillary muscle, as well as to the apex of the heart.

When each site of division of the fiber groups of the left bundle branch of this heart is observed more precisely, in most of the sites — though not always — individual small fiber bundles can be seen extending in various directions, crossing each other just above the angles of division, and forming dense nets. These intercrossings of the small bundles indicate that the fiber elements are not simply divided into two groups, and further that the elements from all parts of a fiber group before division are distributed after division as equally as possible into two fiber groups. For the purpose of equal distribution, some of the fibers situated at the posterior half of the undivided fiber group move to its anterior half just above an angle of division. Inversely, several fibers (bundles of very small and fine fibers) situated at the anterior half also move to the posterior half. In this way, the above-mentioned intercrossing of fibers occurs at the sites of division.

The small groups of muscle fibers very often fuse with each other inferiorly and form reticular nets in a similar way. The nets in the human heart are usually round or oval in shape. The round or oval form of the net angle is due to the above-mentioned intercrossing of the muscle fibers inside the small bundles prior to division. The intercrossing is, of course, not the only reason for the round form of the nets. The peculiar fold formation of the endocardium also contributes to this phenomenon.

In the sheep heart, the terminal ramifications of the connecting bundle are mostly thin fibers, as will be demonstrated later. In contrast, in the human heart they are often broad sheets, frequently covered by endocardium on both sides, and form a very thin membrane. When the ramifications cross over an intertrabecular recess, they often take a membranous form. Not seldom, however, do they take the form of a very small tendinous fiber-like cord, such as seen in the sheep heart. When passing over a recess, broad and flat small muscle bundles converge to form a cord. After passing the recess, the bundles spread again in a fanlike fashion or proceed further in a thin fibrous form in the subendocardium. The ways in which they cross over the intertrabecular recesses are highly variable.

In the left ventricle of the human heart, very long, fine, hair-thin or slightly thicker tendinous fiber-like cords are also seen near the relatively broad muscle fibers. The fine cords are the terminal ramifications of the connecting bundle. Such a cord very often extends from a specific place on the left bundle branch to the posterior or anterior papillary muscle. Often a cord extends from the tip of the posterior papillary muscle upward to the posterosuperior portion of the ventricular septum. (This cord should not be confused with a genuine tendinous fiber. The cord attaches not to the mitral valve, but to the muscular wall. Indeed, it often attaches to various portions of the wall when divided into many twigs.) In addition to these frequently visible cords in specific locations, free cords are occasionally observed at the posterior wall or at the apex of the heart, where trabeculations are well developed. These cords connect relatively remote walls, extending, for example, from one trabeculation to another. Furthermore, they extend from the posterior papillary muscle groups to the adjacent portions of the ventricular wall. In all hearts, the number of fine short cords stretching between two neighboring trabeculations or between the papillary muscles and the adjacent trabeculations is varied.

Macroscopic Observations of the Right Bundle Branch[*]

The inner surface of the right ventricle of the human heart shows great variations, especially in terms of the degree of trabecular development and the number, position and size of the papillary muscles. A relatively smooth portion of the inner surface usually can be seen around the small medial papillary muscle and below the supraventricular crest. This smooth portion soon connects with many trabeculations lower down. On the other hand, the other parts of the wall, namely the ventricular septum and the parietal wall, always show very strong unevenness. At the anterior ventricular septum below the aortic orifice and the medial papillary muscle, there are usually several big trabeculations which extend parallel to each other and vertically

---

[*]For an example, refer to Plate II, Fig. 1.

downward to the parietal wall. (For this description, the heart should be regarded as being in an upright position, with the cardiac base at the top and the apex at the bottom.) The trabeculations do not extend along the transition from the septum to the parietal wall, but rather extend straight across the transition. After reaching the parietal wall, they divide into many smaller trabeculations. In most cases, the posterior ventricular septum is very uneven because many small or big trabeculations extend vertically, or because of the presence of small inconstant papillary muscles. The parietal wall is occupied by numerous trabeculations which generally converge from the cardiac base to the apex and, by joining together, form a net. The medial papillary muscle is found beneath the supraventricular crest, usually as a very small process. An additional one or two small papillary muscles can also exist there on an oblique line in the direction of the posteroinferior area. The anterior papillary muscle is anchored mainly on the parietal wall, near the border between the lower and middle thirds of the transitional line that extends from the septum to the parietal wall. As a rule, this muscle has a supporting trabecular leg that originates at the septum. The leg is sometimes thick and sometimes thin. Rarely is it absent. Where it is absent, usually a trabeculation that extends from below the medial papillary muscle to the parietal wall is connected with the base of the anterior papillary muscle. A clear fusion line can be noted at the site of the connection. The anterior papillary muscle is usually big, and is composed of a long conical process. Rarely, there may be two or three separate papillary muscles. The posterior papillary muscle group usually consists of two or three papillary muscles closely related to each other. They are seated at the posterior recess, where the trabeculations usually run in a most complicated fashion. The legs of the papillary muscles attach partly to the septum and partly to the parietal wall. Knowledge of this anatomical arrangement of the inner surface of the right ventricle is necessary for properly describing the right bundle branch.

It is not always easy in the human heart to identify macroscopically the course of the right bundle branch. Sometimes, the stem of the right bundle branch is even missing. When many hearts are examined carefully, nevertheless, the course can be recognized in several hearts.

The stem of the right bundle branch usually is macroscopically visible near the posterosuperior area of the medial papillary muscle. It appears as a relatively opaque and fine longitudinally fibered endocardial striation. Its width is 1–2 mm in big hearts, and can be 3 mm in certain sites. From its origin, the right bundle branch extends inferiorly and slightly anteriorly, then gradually proceeds inferiorly and posteriorly with a mild or occasionally acute curve. Extending along the above-mentioned supporting trabecular leg, it finally reaches the base of the anterior papillary muscle, where it divides into many twigs which spread in various directions, either along the trabeculations or through the small tendinous fiber-like cords that are especially well suited for this purpose.

The terminal ramifications are directed partly toward the parietal wall and partly toward the ventricular septum. They are usually easy to recognize at the parietal wall, especially in a big hypertrophic heart. At the parietal wall, they extend as relatively wide (1–2 mm) and somewhat elevated strands beneath the endocardium, running either along or obliquely across the trabeculations. They connect with each other and form a relatively large network. The network spreads all over the inner surface of the parietal wall and extends up to the ventricular septum. At some places, however, the terminal ramifications form a wide muscle bundle. When the strands (cords) cross the intertrabecular deep grooves, they extend across them either as round strands of that thickness of hairs or as thin membranes, keeping their former shape as seen in the left bundle branch. After reaching the other side of the grooves, they extend further on in the subendocardium.

If the heart is severely hypertrophied and dilated, the trabeculations are usually also very big and round, and lie in various layers one upon the other. Accordingly, the intertrabecular grooves are sometimes very deep and large. In such cases, the terminal ramifications of the connecting bundle can readily be observed, extending not only along the superficial trabeculations but also toward the deeper ones.

In the ventricular septum, these terminal ramifications are not usually seen as clearly as in the parietal wall. However, in the posterior half of the septum, where the trabeculations are well developed and where many papillary muscles exist, the findings can be made as described above. In particular, one can observe several terminal ramifications extending from the base of the anterior papillary muscle to the posterior papillary muscle group. Furthermore, numerous short or long tendinous fiber-like cords can be seen at the posterior recess, i.e. at the area surrounding the posterior papillary muscles. These cords spread either between two neighboring or somewhat remote trabeculations, or between the papillary muscles, or between a papillary muscle and the neighboring trabeculation. A small number of cords are also found at other places on the septum, especially at the anterior tranisition between the septum and the parietal wall.

As described thus far, the terminal ramifications of the connecting bundle in the human heart generally can be recognized macroscopically with varying difficulty, and can be easily seen in several human hearts. The left bundle branch extends as a very broad and thin bundle, but its course varies considerably from heart to heart. In the human heart, as in all other animal hearts that I examined, approximately one-half of the muscle fibers extend to the anterior and to the posterior papillary muscle, and most of the remaining fibers spread to the apex of the heart. Terminal ramifications, such as those observed in the right ventricle, also exist in the ventricular wall beneath the mitral valve. They originate at the posterior papillary muscle, and do not extend directly from the left bundle branch. This mode of spreading of terminal ramification is similar to that of other mammalian hearts. In the human heart, however, the width of the left bundle branch is usually wider than seen in ungulates (see Plates I and II).

The mode of spreading seen in the right bundle branch of the human heart, therefore, accords strongly with that of other mammalian hearts. What I must emphasize, nonetheless, is that in the human heart several cords which I described in the sheep and dog hearts do not exist. For example, I did not find in the human heart a particular cord, forming an important pathway of the right bundle branch that, in other mammalian hearts, spread from the vicinity of the anterior papillary muscle directly to the parietal wall. In the human heart, the terminal ramifications extend through various trabeculations to the parietal wall. They begin at the base of the anterior papillary muscle and then spread in many directions.

I would like to make one final comment. Until now, only one author, Henle, has insisted that Purkinje fibers can be seen macroscopically in the human heart. He stated that Purkinje fibers appear as gray fibers only in the first month of life. This view was adopted in many textbooks. In order to confirm his view, I precisely examined young hearts. However, I could never find macroscopically such a fiber in the small hearts. In contrast, as described above, I could always find these fibers with more or less facility in big hearts. If it was true that Henle observed Purkinje fibers in young hearts, he ought to have seen them even more readily in big hearts. He did not describe any exact microscopic findings relating to the fibers. Probably he did not perform any microscopic examinations. If he had performed them, he would have reported the results, because so far all previous investigators have failed to recognize Purkinje fibers in the human heart. I can now say with certainty that the histological characteristics of Purkinje fibers in the human are quite different from those of the ungulates. Henle, therefore, apparently made some error. Probably he thought that small trabeculations or tendinous fibers were Purkinje fibers, and other authors accepted Henle's statement without verifying its accuracy by conducting their own examinations.

Gegenbauer stated that Purkinje fibers were definitely found microscopically not only in the endocardium but also within the myocardium of the heart of a 15-year-old human being. Strangely, he did not present detailed findings either, and only stated that the fibers were the same as the "well-known" Purkinje fibers. I am convinced that the human heart contains no such Purkinje fibers as he described. Instead, the muscle fibers of the terminal ramification in the human are totally different histologically from the "well-known" Purkinje fibers. Gegenbauer's statement, therefore, must also have been based upon an error.

(c) *Cat heart*

(1) *No. 150. The adult cat heart*

As usual, the cardiac septal wall was sectioned horizontally at 9-micron thickness from top to bottom, the sectioning being approximately parallel to the line of closure of the aortic valve. Every eighth section was retained for investigation.

In section No. 21, for the first time a peculiaar muscle group can be seen which is situated beneath the joining point of the right coronary and noncoronary aortic leaflets, being located at the uppermost portion of the ventricular septum. On the left, it is bordered by the endocardium and the thick connective tissue of the original portion of the aorta. On the right, it

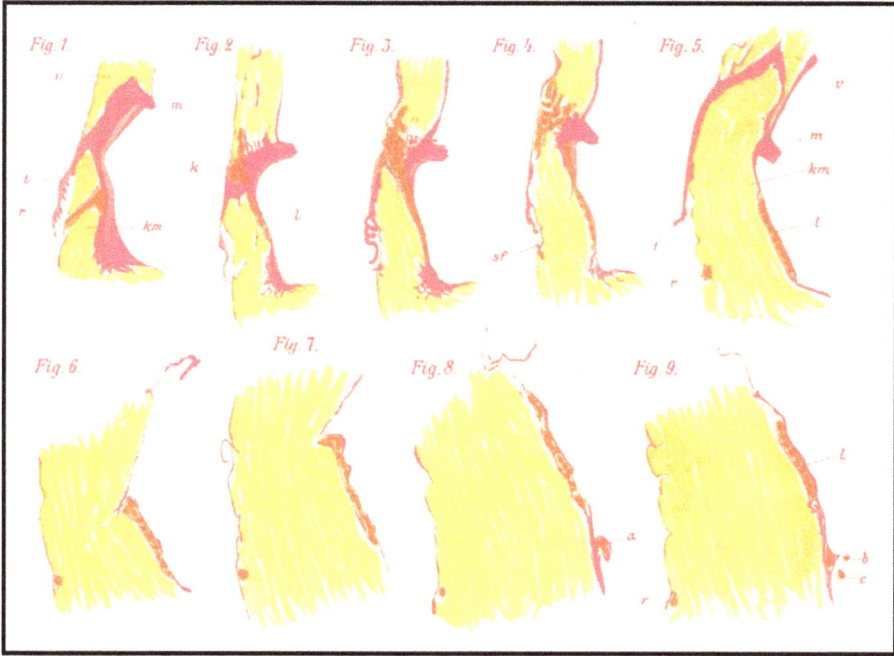

Cat heart No. 150

v, k, s, m, t, km, l and r are the same as for human heart No. 139

a = part of muscle fibers of the left bundle branch enters a small tendinous fiber-like cord, which is soon divided into two smaller cords (b and c)

sf = tendinous fiber for the septal leaflet of the tricuspid valve

is bordered by musculature of the ventricular septum. The muscle group is also separated by connective tissue from the septal musculature. In the next section, it becomes much larger, is elongated with a tip to the right and anteriorly, and almost reaches the right side endocardium (Fig. 1 = section No. 22). At the same time, it elongates somewhat to the left and anteriorly. It is, therefore, divided into the right and left bundle branches. In the subsequent sections, the right bundle branch goes further anteriorly and loses it posterior connection to the main mass which rapidly elongates anteriorly in the subendocardium (i.e. it becomes the left bundle branch).

In section No. 25, a characteristically stained muscle group appears in the atrium, nestling close to the right side of the atrioventricular fibrous septum. It contains numerous nuclei, mostly oval and compact, and consists of much more slender and less clearly differentiated fibers than those of the ordinary atrial musculature. Each fiber of this muscle group runs quite irregularly, combines with each other and forms a complicated glomerular network. In the next section, the muscle group moves anteriorly and somewhat leftward, and its anterior tip reaches the atrioventricular fibrous septum (Fig. 2 = section No. 26). In the next two sections, the muscle group penetrates the septum, approaches the left bundle branch mentioned above, and connects with this bundle branch. In the sections which follow, it is then separated from the left bundle branch (Figs. 3 and 4 = sections No. 28 and No. 32). In this case, the atrial segment of the atrioventricular connecting bundle can still be seen until section No. 48 and its extension is relatively broad. It extends posteriorly up to the coronary sinus and anteriorly up to the line of attachment of the septal leaflet of the tricuspid valve. The atrial segment of the bundle has more, and stronger, connective tissue between individual muscle fibers or between individual muscle groups than in the ordinary atrial musclature, especially at its transition to the latter. Here, at certain places of this transition, there exists a sharp border of connective tissue. At other places, there is no clear border, and there are only scattered strong connective tissue fibers. It seemed to me as if the connecting bundle gradually connected here with the ordinary atrial musculature by losing its strong interstitial connective tissue and, at the same time, changing its histological characteristics, thus aquiring the characteristics of the ordinary atrial muscle fibers.

As stated above, the right bundle branch, after approaching rapidly the endocardium, runs far anteroinferiorly separated from the endocardium by a small amount of ventricular muscle fibers. The bundle gradually becomes smaller (for example, in section No. 56, the cross-section is 0.8 × 0.3 mm; on the other hand, in section No. 136, it is 0.3 × 0.25 mm). As its connective tissue component is minimal, I could only follow the bundle inferiorly by noting its slight staining differences, by the rich connective tissue between each fiber, and through careful serial tracing of the bundle to distinguish it from the adjacent septal musculature. In van Gieson preparations, the connecting bundle is stained somewhat more pale and red, whereas the ordinary musculature is stained rather yellow or brown. Finally, the right bundle branch reaches directly the subendocardium and runs like a bridge along a big trabecular muscle which extends from the septum to the base of the anterior papillary muscle. I could not then follow it distally any more.

At the beginning, the left bundle branch runs horizontally for a short distance forward and somewhat downward. The muscle fibers of the bundle branch are numerous, but they gradually reduce their number as traced downward. The direction of the bundle branch becomes more vertical. During its downward course, the position shifts somewhat anteriorly but it always stays in the subendocardium. In section No. 56, its horizontal width is about 4 mm. The individual fibers are here sectioned transversely or obliquely and become scattered in fine subencocardial connective tissue fibers. Connecting with each other, the individual fibers form a large meshed net and the mesh is filled with connective tissue (Fig. 5 = section No. 56). In this fashion, the left bundle branch runs almost vertically downward. On the way, the amount of the fibers increases to some extent but then again decreases (Fig. 6 = section No. 80). In section No. 104 = Fig. 7, it is roughly divided into two groups, which, however, are not extensive (the width is about 6 mm in section No. 104). In the subsequent sections, some of the fibers gradually go in groups into fine tendinous fiber-like cords and leave the endocardium. Thus, the remaining fibers in the subendocardium, running further downward, become more and more sparse. This preparation ended here, about 1 cm below the lowest attachment of the noncoronary aortic leaflet (Figs. 8 and 9 = sections No. 136 and No. 142). Up to here, the bundle branch always runs in a closed bundle, though loose. I cannot say with certainty whether these fibers already connected with the ordinary cardiac musculature. This is because the histological characteristics of both muscle elements became similar and, for this reason, I could not differentiate them, especially in the lower area of this preparation. At any rate, I am sure that connections between the two muscle elements are extremely rare, even if they ever happen, because up to here both elements are separated always by varying amounts of connective tissue.

(2) *No. 151 and No. 154. The cat hearts*

In these two serial preparations of the cat hearts, which were, as with the previous preparation No. 150, sectioned horizontally parallel to the connecting line of the lowest attachments of the noncoronary and right coronary aortic leaflets, I generally recognized the same findings as described for the previous preparation, but I also recognized several variations in each specimen.

In these hearts, it was the atrial segment of the atrioventricular connecting bundle that appeared first, as was always the case in the hearts of ungulates when sectioned in the same way. I might have unintentionally sectioned heart No. 150 somewhat obliquely, so that in the sections of this heart I recognized the initial portion of the left and right bundle branchs before the atrial segment.

In hearts No. 150 and No. 151, the atrial segment of the bundle stretched posteriorly up to the coronary sinus, but in heart No. 154, it did not reach there.

The thickness of the bundle was not the same in all the cat hearts. For example, the portion dividing into the two bundle branches and the initial portion of both the bundle branches were much thicker in heart No. 154 than in hearts No. 150 and No. 151. The right bundle branch in No. 154 was, therefore, seen very clearly, whereas that in heart No. 151 was so weak that I could trace it only several millimeters.

(3) *No. 156. The cat heart*

In this heart, I sectioned horizontally the left ventricle, cutting vertical to the cardiac axis, serially from top to bottom in 9-micron thickness, and each 14th section was retained, in order to investigate the extent of the spread of the atrioventricular connecting bundle in the left ventricle. The sections were stained first with Haematoxylin and then with van Gieson. To reduce the size of the object, the left ventricular peripheral wall of the septum was cut away as much as possible.

By thorough examination of the sections, the left bundle branch can first be seen running downward in a relatively wide but thin and loose bundle from beneath the middle point of the connecting line of the lowest attachments of the right coronary and noncoronary aortic leaflets, as already described for the other cat heart (No. 150). These fibers, however, are not recognized anywhere other than here at this level of the wall. For the first time at the anterior septum, 1–2 mm beneath the attachment of the anterior mitral leaflet, above the tip of the anterior papillary muscle, several special muscle groups are recognized subendocardially, which seem to have no relation either to each other or to the left bundle branch. The muscle fibers lie scattered in subendocardial loose connective tissue and stain somewhat paler than the adjacent cardiac musculature. They are sectioned sometimes transversely and sometimes longitudinally. By examining further inferiorly, numerous similar subendocardial muscle fibers are seen to appear in various parts of the wall.

When each of the muscle groups is traced, it can be recognized in most cases that the muscle groups connect at a somewhat lower level with a small tendinous fiber-like cord stretching through the ventricular chamber, or combine first with one of the other similar muscle groups and connect through the latter with a tendinous fiber-like cord. When the course of these cords is further followed, it is found that the cords form a net in the ventricle, combining together or ramifying with each other in many ways. The above-mentioned muscle groups, therefore, exist not as isolated islands but related to each other in the subendocardium or through the cords.

The stem of the left bundle branch runs about 5 mm downward without any change and then is gradually divided in the subendocardium into two groups, i.e. the anterior and the posterior division. After running about 2 mm further downward, the main mass of the anterior division enters a tendinous fiber-like cord and its small remaining mass of the fibers runs further downward in the subendocardium. A portion of the muscle fibers of the posterior division enters, somewhat further below, another tendinous fiber-like cord. Both of these cords ramify in many twigs in the ventricle and, combining and dividing in many ways, form a complicated network during their courses. The remaining portion of the muscle fibers of the posterior division in the subendocardium runs further downward and enters a tendinous fiber-like cord. Ramifying in twigs, it connects with other cords and contributes to the formation of a net, which is nothing but part of the larger and more extensive net. Numerous peripheral cords of the network attach to various portions of the ventricular wall, partly by extending back upward to the cardiac base but mostly by extending to the anterior and posterior papillary muscles. From all these attachments, the muscle fibers spread further in the subendocardium. These subendocardial terminal ramifications are the same as the muscle fibers mentioned earlier. It is very interesting to pursue microscopically how individual cords run in the ventricular cavity and connect with each other, and how they ramify or attach to the wall, releasing there their contents, i.e. the muscle fibers. I cannot describe them in detail, however, because they are much too complicated. In addition, there are numerous short tendinous fiber-like cords which have no direct connection to the network extending through the ventricle. Mostly, they connect adjacent points of the wall. Often they bridge gaps between two neighboring trabeculations, which develop markedly in the cat heart. From my viewpoint, these short cords seem to provide in the shortest possible way rapid spread of the subendocardial terminal ramifications of the atrioventricular connecting bundle. Most of the cords are no thicker than a hair, are rarely thicker and are often much thinner than a hair. Their transverse section is usually round, and often oval or flat. Its surface is covered with endocardium and its subendocardial connective tissue fibers are almost always thick and strong. The muscle fibers usually run in the middle of the cord, but are not infrequently pressed to one side. In smaller cords, the muscle fibers are usually arranged as a small round bundle, surrounded by strong connective tissue fibers. On the other hand, the muscle fibers of relatively large cords are often arranged more or less loosely, penetrated by loose connective tissue. In these circumstances, each muscle fiber does not run in the same direction of the cord but runs relatively curled.

(4) *Macroscopic description*

Surprised by these interesting findings, I examined macroscopically a new cat heart. In this heart, I saw well the formation of nets in the left ventricle. The findings are basically the same as those described for heart No. 156. But I also recognized small differences. This is understandable, if several hearts are macroscopically compared, because the inner surfaces of the ventricles look somewhat different in each heart, especially in terms of development of the trabeculations and the papillary muscles.

In this preparation, I could see macroscopically the upper course of the left bundle branch as a relatively broad and somewhat white gray cord running downward from beneath the right half of the noncoronary aortic leaflet. It divided very early into two groups. About 1.5 mm beneath the connecting line between the lowest attachments of the noncoronary and right coronary aortic leaflets, at the anterior border of the left bundle branch, an about two-hair-width, brown–gray and somewhat elevated cord is seen, running anteroinferiorly in the subendocardium. On the other hand, the remaining flat and broad posterior group runs almost vertically downward. At about 5 mm beneath the lowest attachment of the right coronary aortic leaflet, this anterior division gradually becomes distinct inferiorly and, while dividing into two twigs, gradually leaves the suebendocardium and enters the ventricular cavity in the form of two cords. These cords run down and diverge, dividing into many twigs, and form a network by dividing and connecting with each other. Finally, most of the cords of the network attach to various parts of the anterior papillary muscle, whilst the remaining cords attach to various parts of the wall near the anterior papillary muscle and to the apex of the heart.

The broad posterior division of the left bundle branch runs downward without initially giving off any special cords. For the first time, at about 6 mm beneath the aortic valve, several cords arise from its posterior border. They mainly run to the posterior papillary muscle, giving forth many additional twigs on their way, whilst its anterior half first gives forth very fine cords more inferiorly. All these cords and their numerous twigs repeatedly connect and divide, forming a network which also connects with the above-mentioned network. The meshes of the network are sometimes large and sometimes small, the sizes of the meshes being variable. The thickness of the fibers of the net is also variable; they are rarely two hairs thick, sometimes one hair thick and not infrequently as large as wool hair. As already stated above, many fine fibers run not only to the papillary muscles but also to various parts of the inner wall from various points of the network, especially from its periphery. Distinct deposits of fat are frequently recognizable at the attachments of the fine fibers, which are mainly seen at the lower half of the ventricle. Except for the above-mentioned initial portion of the left bundle branch and the free cords in the ventricle, no special subendocardial fibers were seen macroscopically in this preparation.

Such a free net was not recognized in the right ventricle, and the right bundle branch of the atioventricular connecting bundle was not macroscopically visible. Furthermore, in this heart, there was a relatively thick but short muscle trabeculation which, arising from the ventricular septum, ran directly to the base of the anterior papillary muscle through the ventricular chamber, and usually led the right bundle branch of the connecting bundle to the papillary muscle. The anterior papillary muscle, therefore, has a second base besides its ordinary base on the parietal wall. Very fine, short cords mostly only of the thickness of wool hair, which bridged the gaps between the trabeculations or bridged the anterior and posterior transitions of the ventricular septum to the parietal wall, were fairly frequently seen, especially at the latter sites.

(d) *Sheep heart*

(1) *No. 155. The sheep heart*

In the examination of these serial preparations, several longitudinally sectioned muscle fibers or muscle fiber bundles are seen on the dorsal site of the initial sections, namely near the coronary sinus and at its upper border. Here and there, the muscle fibers, or the bundles of muscle fibers, combine with each other to form nets. On the other hand, the neighboring atrial musculature is exclusively sectioned transversely. Histologically, these longitudinally sectioned muscle fibers seem not to differ from the atrial musculature. In the following sections, the net formations become more and more apparent. In the beginning, the meshes of the nets are large, while they later become smaller. The more or less round meshes are filled with transversely sectioned muscle fibers, or else with fatty tissue, nerve bundles and loose connective tissue fibers. The muscle fibers forming these networks come and go in various directions. Their main direction, however, is toward the right, downward or toward the left, and they connect with the ordinary atrial muscle fibers. Fatty tissue gradually increases inferiorly, especially on the left side of the network, so that the fatty tissue compresses almost all the muscle tissue and only scattered muscle fibers run through the fatty tissue (f) as branches of the network toward the left or inferiorly.

In section No. 31, a peculiar muscle mass (k) appears on the left side of the above-mentioned network, between the network and the fatty tissue (f).

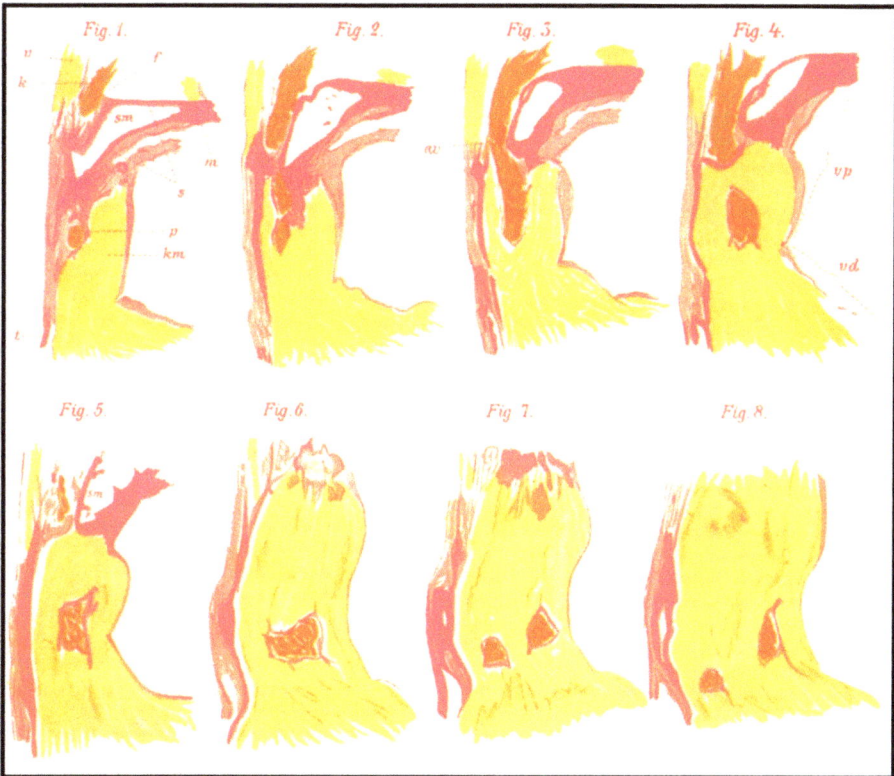

Sheep heart No. 155

v, k, s, m, t and *km* are the same as for human heart No. 139

      p = initial portion of the ventricular bundle

     av = penetrating canal of the connecting bundle through the atrioventricular septum

     vp = area of the noncoronary leaflet of the aortic valve

     vd = area of the right coronary leaflet of the aortic valve

     sm = bone marrow in the atrioventricular septum

   l & *r* = the left and the right bundle branch of the connecting system

Figure 11 indicates how Purkinje fibers exist in a long intraventricular tendinous fiber-like cord which is not a valvar tendinous fiber. Illustration *A* shows the initial portion of the tendinous fiber-like cord in which four Purkinje fibers of different sizes are visible. They are divided into many smaller fibers in a further course (*B*). Further distally, the cord is divided into three cords (*C, D* and *E*). Also, Purkinje fibers enter individual cords. Until now, such cords have been erroneously called abnormal tendinous fibers in the ventricular cavity and mistaken for either congenital malformation of the heart or pathological products.

(*continued on next page*)

(*continued from previous page*)

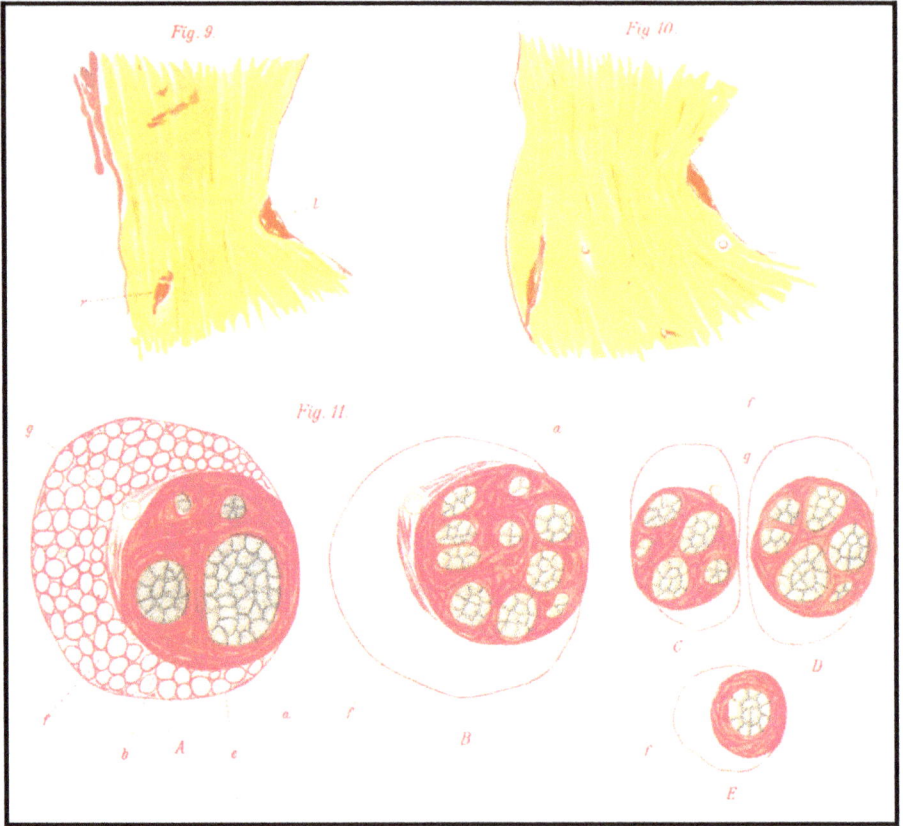

a = a cross-sectioned Purkinje fiber
b = thick connective tissue
e = endocardial layer
f = characteristic fatty capsule of the cord
g = blood vessel

The mass is characterized by its fine fibers, its abundance of nuclei and its very complicated irregular netlike arrangement. The fine fibers are directly connected with the large fibers of the above-mentioned network. In the following sections, this group of peculiar muscle fibers becomes gradually larger and the connection between this and the large fiber network constantly decreases as fatty tissue appears between them (sections No. 31–37). In section No. 38, most of this network of fine fibers lies in the fatty tissue (f), so that its connection with the network of large fibers is no more seen, because there is only a small amount of the network of large fibers here. In the next section, the network of fine fibers (k) rapidly elongates and enlarges anteriorly toward the atrioventricular fibrocartilaginous septum (s), which extends obliquely from the base of the aortic leaflet of the mitral valve (m) lying to the left and posteriorly to the base of the septal leaflet of the tricuspid valve (t) lying to the right and anteriorly. This septum is mainly made up of bone tissue in the sheep heart. The bony septum shows a hollow at the place corresponding to the anterior tip of the network of fine fibers (k) (Fig. 1 = section No. 39). In section No. 40, this hollow rapidly grows and the muscle group of the network moves its head into the hollow. At the same time, the posterior part of the muscle group gradually reduces its size. The muscle group suddenly shows a highly remarkable change at the place of its entrance into the hollow. The fibers of this muscle groups had been very fine before, forming an entirely irregular and highly complicated thick plexus. At the entrance to the hollow, this network of fine fibers connects with a quite peculiar tissue (p), which is a net composed of highly irregular and varying-formed large and usually polyhedral cells. The individual cells have one or two, seldom three, nuclei and show relatively sparse and much less regular longitudinal and unclear cross stripes even when compared to primitive cardiac muscle fibers. The protoplasmic mass of the cells is very rich and somewhat transparent, though not homogeneous. These peculiar cells make groups by joining at their front and rear, or side by side, forming various-sized cords. These cords again combine with each other and form an irregular network. The connection between this and the above-mentioned network of small fibers is relatively simple. From the network of large cells originate many small fibers with fibrils. Thus, direct connection occurs between the two networks.

In section No. 39, at a small area in the ventricular portion, this network of large cells (*p*) is already seen, adhering close to the atrioventricular cartilaginous septum (*s*) and confronting the network of small fibers in the atrium. In the next preparation, this large cell structure in the ventricle enlarges and elongates posteriorly against the cartilaginous septum. As a result, the cartilaginous septum has a new hollow. In section No. 41, the anterior and posterior hollows in the septum become deeper and, in section No. 42, the septum is penetrated, thus forming a canal. The anterior and posterior networks of large cells combine in this canal and a connection between the atrium and the ventricle is established by this peculiar bundle of large cells (Fig. 2 = section No. 41). The network of small fibers in the atrium becomes bigger, and the connections between this and the ordinary atrial musculature are quite sparse. On the other hand, the connection between this and the network of large cells becomes more prominent, reaching its highest degree in sections No. 43–45. The network of small fibers is largest in sections No. 43 and No. 44. Here, the horizontal width is about 1.2 mm and the anteroposterior length is about 4 mm. It extends forward just up to the entrance of the canal (Fig. 3 = section No. 44). In the sections which follow, this network gradually becomes smaller, being penetrated by strong or fine connective tissues, before disappearing entirely in section No. 50. The network is always separated by a layer of atrial musculature 1–2 mm thick from the right-side endocardium of the atrial septum.

The peculiar bundle of large cells (*p*), which is the continuation of the network of small cells (*k*) in the atrial septum, gradually becomes larger from section No. 39, and occupies the entire canal of the atrioventricular fibrocartilaginous septum in section No. 42. It gradually extends forward and breaks into the ventricular musculature (*km*). The individual cell cords, or cell processes, which together constitute the bundle or the network, are surrounded like a sheath by thick or thin connective tissue fibers. Loose connective tissue fibers and fatty tissues are also seen sparsely in the meshes. In the course of serial sections, the posterior of the bundle is seen to be gradually strangulated by connective tissue and, in section No. 47 (Fig. 4), the network of large cells is completely separated from the network of small cells, which is still visible in the atrium. Now, the network of large cells lies entirely in the ventricular septum. It does not run horizontally and anteriorly as before, but inferiorly and slightly anteriorly.

This is because here the individual cords of the network are cut no more longitudinally but mostly obliquely and, therefore, the sectional form of the bundle is no more longitudinal posteroanteriorly but is irregularly oval. Here, the bundle composed of the network of large cells runs just in the middle of the ventricular septum. In other words, the bundle lies the same distance from both the left and the right endocardium and, in this position, gradually runs anteroinferiorly. The thickness of the bundle gradually increases. As stated above, all the cell cords are surrounded by connective tissue sheaths, and the entire complex of cell cords is also surrounded by a common connective tissue sheath, forming a bundle as a whole. Thus, the bundle is completely separated by the sheath from the surrounding ordinary ventricular musculature. Twigs of connective tissue of the sheath are connected with the intramuscular connective tissues. At the beginning, the horizontal sectional form of the bundle is somewhat longer in its posteroanterior direction than in its width. Later, the length–width relation gradually becomes inverted. In section No. 58, the cut shape is oval. In this section, the transverse diameter is about 3 mm and the posteroanterior diameter is about 2 mm (Figs. 5 and 6 = sections No. 49 and No. 58).

In the next section, No. 59, the bundle is divided into two groups, the left and the right, by connective tissue appearing at the middle of the bundle in the posteroanterior direction. In the following sections, the two groups very rapidly move away from each other in closed bundles.

The left bundle branch, i.e. the left group, is somewhat larger than the right and more rapidly approaches the left endocardium. Already in section No. 68, it reaches the left endocardium. The course of the bundle branch is almost vertically downward, and it is directed slightly anteriorly. On its way, the characteristics of the individual cells gradually change. The cells gradually become paler and more homogenous as the bundle proceeds downward, and show the almost typical appearance of the well-known Purkinje cells as the bundle approaches the left endocardium. The number of the cells, as well as the thickness of the left bundle branch, varies according to the level of the section. The cell cords usually take the same direction as that of the bundle branch. Here, almost all the cords, which are composed of numerous cells, are therefore sectioned crosswise. The sectional form of the individual cords is quite manifold. Some are round and others are longish and oval, bean-formed, indented and so on.

This indicates that, here, the cell cords do not show a beautiful round shape and do not run parallelling each other, as seen in the lower course of the bundle branch, as we will see later. But this indicates that the cords have irregular shapes, run obliquely in varied degrees, and form a network of relatively short meshes by connecting with each other. So far, the left bundle branch is always sharply separated from the adjacent cardiac musculature by a connective tissue sheath and there is no connection between them (Figs. 7 and 8 = sections No. 60 and No. 65).

In the next sections subendocardial connective tissue fibers connect with the sheath of the left bundle branch and the left bundle branch partly loses its own sheath. Numerous connective tissue fibers coming from the relatively thick subendocardial connective tissue penetrate between each cell cord of the left bundle branch, and no special laminar sheath separates the bundle branch from the endocardium. The individual cell cords still have their own individual connective tissue sheaths and, likewise, a sharp connective tissue sheath exists between the right side of the bundle branch and the ordinary cardiac musculature. Up to now, the cell cords frequently combine with each other by crosswise or obliquely running cell cords and are arranged more or less in a reticular formation. Now, they do not combine with each other so often, but run more independently and parallelly. The number of the cell cords gradually decreases, but the size of each cord increases somewhat. The crosswise section of each cord is mostly round, and each cord usually contains 3–10 cells, lying side by side. Each of the cells already shows the well-known beautiful characteristics of Purkinje fibers. Usually, the peripheral portion of the cells is roughly granulated or somewhat striped. The center, on the other hand, shows an entirely homogenous appearance. They contain one or two, seldom three, nuclei which usually lie in a bright halo. All the bundles of the left bundle branch lie completely in the subendocardium and its crosswise section is a longish oval. In section No. 74, the horizontal subendocardial width is about 2.5 mm and the thickness is 0.7 mm. Here, the bundle is composed of roughly 50 cell cords or Purkinje fibers (Fig. 9 = section No. 74).

In the following sections, fibers of the connective tissue separating the left bundle branch from the neighboring cardiac musculature gradually come into a closer relationship with intrafascicular connective tissue fibers of the adjacent cardiac musculature. Many twigs of the connective tissue fibers separating the bundle branch from the cardiac musculature enter the cardiac muscle and connect with its connective tissues. The characteristic large cell cords, however, have no connection with the cardiac musculature. They run as a closed bundle further downward along the endocardium. In section No. 85, a tiny cord of large cells leaves for the first time the subendocardial connective tissue surrounding the left bundle branch and slowly enters the cardiac musculature, running downward surrounded by cardiac musculature on all sides. But it slowly returns to its former course without connecting with the ordinary cardiac musculature and, in section No. 97, it takes a place in the subendocardial connective tissue near the bundle branch. (At this section, this serial preparation ended approximately 1 cm beneath the lowest attachment of the aortic valvar leaflet. The left bundle branch will be followed further in the other preparation, after the upper course of the right bundle branch is described from this preparation.)

In section No. 59, the right bundle branch runs almost vertically downward and somewhat anteriorly after separating from the left bundle branch. In the sections which follow, it gradually becomes smaller, whereas the left bundle branch becomes larger. In section No. 68, it is only half as large as the left bundle branch. It gradually approaches the right endocardium. In section No. 68, however, it does not reach the right endocardium, whilst the left bundle branch already reaches the left endocardium. The structure of the right bundle branch is generally the same as that of the left bundle branch. It also has a connective tissue sheath and is entirely separated from the adjacent cardiac musculature. When the right bundle branch is compared with the left bundle branch at the same height, it is noteworthy that there is a definite difference in the character of each cell constituting the right bundle branch in which the cells combine together side by side or one after another. Each cell of the left bundle branch changes its characteristics gradually but relatively rapidly by becoming homogenous after separating from the right. In contrast, the characteristics of the cells of the right bundle branch change much more slowly. Therefore, if the two bundle branches are compared in the same section, for example in section No. 68, a great difference in staining intensity can be recognized. Here, the cells of the left bundle branch are stained in a pale and unclear fashion, but those of the right bundle branch are stained relatively opaque and yellow–brown. This is the reason why the cell border of the right bundle branch is not as clearly recognized as that of the left bundle branch.

In the subsequent sections, the form of each cell cord seems gradually to become regularly rounded. Here, the crosswise but somewhat oblique section of the cell cord looks, therefore, mostly oval. The numerous irregular connections observed before cannot now be seen so often, although branchings and reunifications of the cell cords can still be recognized when the sections are carefully pursued. The cells constituting the cords gradually reduce their staining intensity and, in section No. 80, show the typical appearance of Purkinje fibers. From section No. 73, the form of the horizontal section of the right bundle branch gradually becomes a longish spindle (in section No. 85, the length is about 2.5 mm and the width 0.5 mm). Accordingly, the sectional surface of most of the cell cords is a longish oval. The change of the sectional form indicates that the course of the right bundle branch is now no more vertically downward, but rather anteriorly and somewhat downward. The number of cell cords reduces now but its thickness increases to some extent, as the cell cords are formed of more cells lying crosswise side by side. The right bundle branch still takes a course within the cardiac musculature, 1–0.5 mm away from the right endocardium. All through its course up to now, the right bundle branch is surrounded by a connective tissue sheath and is separated from the adjacent cardiac musculature. Connective tissue fibers of the sheath extend very often as twigs into the adjacent ordinary cardiac muscle bundles and connect with their interstitial connective tissue fibers, or preferentially with vascular connective tissues between the muscles. In section No. 97, this preparation ended as I already stated in the description of the left bundle branch. Before tracing the continuation of the left and right bundle branches in the preparations especially made for this purpose, I also examined other parts of this preparation (No. I) and searched for other Purkinje fibers.

In section No. 15, several transverse sections of very small Purkinje fibers are already seen running in the right subendocardium around the supraventricular crest, the muscle ridge between the tricuspid and pulmonary orifices, and in the transition between the septal and parietal walls. Purkinje fibers most frequently appear inferiorly at various sites, not only subendocardially but also intramuscularly. They very often connect directly with the cardiac musculature in various fashions. They never connect, however, with the right bundle branch running in the very vicinity. It is also noteworthy that Purkinje fibers never extend near the attachment of the septal leaflet of the tricuspid valve. The situation is the same with the left surface of the ventricular septum. Here, small typical Purkinje fibers can be seen scattered for the first time in the subendocardium several millimeters beneath the lowest attachments of the aortic valvar leaflets. Purkinje fibers increase their size and number inferiorly, and appear in the ordinary muscle bundles here and there connecting with the ordinary cardiac muscle fibers. Here, Purkinje fibers have no relationship with the thick left bundle branch running downward in the subendocardium.

Now, I will trace further the course of the right bundle branch using new serial sections made for this purpose from the right half of the ventricular septum. This preparation (No. III) is the direct continuation of preparation No. I. It contains, however, only the right bundle branch. I have separated the left half containing the continuation of the left bundle branch from the right half, and made serial sections which I will describe later. This is because the ventricular septum here was very thick. It was too difficult to make serial sections of the whole septum. Moreover, it seemed to me that it was not necessary to use such a difficult method. From my many previous experiences in examining the hearts of humans, dogs and cats, I was convinced that in the sheep hearts also both of the bundle branches must take their courses in the subendocardium. For these reasons, I cut out a piece of only a 2–3 mm thickness containing the endocardium, fixed it in condensed alcohol, embedded it in paraffin and serially sectioned it, horizontally from top to bottom, at a 9-micron thickness. I regularly took every 12th section from this material, mounted them in series, and stained them first with Haematoxylin and then with van Gieson.

In this preparation (No. III), the right bundle branch is again recognized by its spindle sectional form, as was the case in the last sections of preparation No. I (Fig. 10 = section No. 85-I). The front tip gradually becomes stumplike as the sections proceed and consequently reaches the right subendocardial connective tissue. The sectional form again becomes gradually shorter and more oval. The direction, therefore, now runs more in a downward fashion. It is always surrounded by a relatively thick connective tissue sheath and is sharply separated from the adjacent cardiac musculature. Many fatty tissues appear, here, not only inside but also outside the sheath. Likewise, each of the cell cords is surrounded by its own sheath. The main and subordinate sheaths are very often joined together by connective tissue fibers. After running for a short distance in the subendocardium, the right bundle branch again becomes surrounded by cardiac musculature on all sides, then enters a muscular trabeculation and extends toward the anterior papillary muscle. Here, the right bundle branch is a closed bundle consisting of approximately 20–30 cell cords, or Purkinje fibers, lying close side by side. This muscular trabeculation exists constantly in the sheep hearts. It bridges the right ventricular cavity from a certain site of the septum, about 1.5 cm beneath the supraventricular crest, to the big anterior papillary muscle, usually sitting flat at an anteroinferior portion of the parietal wall. The length and size of the trabeculation vary greatly. The trabeculation is, however, usually 1.5 cm in length and 2 mm in thickness. It is a bundle of cardiac muscle surrounded by the endocardium, with the right bundle branch running in its axis. From my viewpoint, therefore, the muscle bundle is nothing but a bridge permitting the right bundle branch to reach the anterior papillary muscle through a shorter way than passing round the corner of the transition from the septum to the parietal wall. Similar circumstances are frequently seen in humans and other animals. Preparation No. III ended at about one half of the length of the trabeculation.

Now, I sectioned in series the anterior papillary muscle with the trabeculation and further studied the course of the right bundle branch. In this preparation, I confirmed that the right bundle branch ran to the base of the papillary muscle as a closed bundle, always surrounded by a connective tissue sheath. Just after reaching the papillary muscle, the bundle was divided into many twigs and spread in various directions, mostly in the subendocardium but partly within the myocardium. Here, I would like to mention a remarkable fact that a very fine tendinous fiber-like cord, approximately 2 cm long but of horsehair thickness, originated from the anterior papillary muscle and extended toward the posterior papillary muscle through the right ventricular cavity. From the already mentioned terminal ramifications of the right bundle branch, a single cell cord (Purkinje fiber) entered this cord and ran to the posterior papillary muscle. During its course, this cord sent a short twig also containing a single cell cord to the septum.

It was impossible for me microscopically to trace the further course of each terminal ramification of the right bundle branch, because the ramifications ran in far too complicated a manner. I will later describe macroscopically these terminal ramifications.

In preparation No. III, as in preparation No. I, numerous Purkinje fibers were seen sectioned mostly in a crosswise fashion, and seldom obliquely or lengthwise in the subendocardium, running in all possible directions within the myocardium. These Purkinje fibers connected directly with the ordinary cardiac musculature in various places not only subendocardially but also at a deeper muscular layer of the septum. *Especially remarkable is the fact that the right bundle branch, whose cells already showed before the typical characteristics of the well-known Purkinje fibers, neither gave any single twig nor connected with the adjacent cardiac muscle fibers but ran entirely isolated. Only after reaching the anterior papillary muscle did the right bundle branch unfastened itself as the terminal ramifications.* Even those Purkinje fibers existing very near the relatively big right bundle branch in the above-mentioned trabeculation also stayed isolated from the bundle branch (even when they ran so close to it).

Now, I will further trace the course of the left bundle branch, using preparation No. IV, which is a direct continuation of preparation No. I. As I mentioned in the case of preparation No. I, the left bundle branch already ran relatively downward as a rather wide bundle in the subendocardium without connecting with the adjacent cardiac musculature. In the initial several sections of preparation No. IV, the course is all but the same as in the last sections of preparation No. I (Fig. 10). It runs further downward in the subendocardium and gradually widens both anteriorly and posteriorly. Fatty tissues gradually appear abundantly between each cell cord of the bundle. At the same time, several fine connective tissues from the endocardium enter, through cell cords, the cardiac musculature. The sheath of the bundle (or, more exactly, connective tissue fibers between the bundle and the cardiac musculature, as there is no proper sheath surrounding the bundle) gradually becomes thinner and less clear. Therefore, both elements, i.e. the ventricular muscle fibers and Purkinje fibers, come close to each other and sometimes run mixed together at certain sites, especially at the boundary. They are, however, always separated from each other by variable connective tissue fibers, so that no direct connection between the two can be found. The course of the cell cords is directed vertically from above to below, because up to now each of the cell cords is almost exclusively cut crosswise. The number of cell cords in the left bundle branch varies considerably, as is also the case with the right bundle branch, depending upon the extent of division or union of the cell cords (sections No. 1–25).

In the subsequent sections, the subendocardial horizontal width of the bundle becomes larger (for example, it is about 4.5 mm in section No. 29), whilst the thickness becomes somewhat reduced. In the next sections, sectional forms of cell cords of the anterior half of the bundle become gradually more oblique or even longish. The direction of the bundle, therefore, now bends anteriorly. In section No. 45, this anterior group is seen to be separated and very distant from the main bundle, and then the cell cords gradually become again sectioned in a crosswise fashion (therefore, they run vertically downward). In this way, the left bundle branch is now divided into two groups. At this level, a new phenomenon is observed. A small cell cord (Purkinje fiber) of the left bundle branch runs into the muscular layer, accompanied by connective tissue coming partly from the subendocardial connective tissue and partly from the interstitial connective tissue of the septal musculature. It runs irregularly upward and branches into many fine twigs. The final twigs connect with the adjacent ordinary muscle fibers (sections No. 26–45). In the further course downward, such a phenomenon like this, i.e. a direct connection between the two elements in the subendocardium, is very seldom observed.

The two divisions of the left bundle branch gradually separate from each other. The larger posterior division runs vertically downward as a continuation of the main bundle. On the other hand, the smaller anterior division runs somewhat anteriorly downward.

The anterior division shows a characteristic change during its further course: the subendocardial connective tissue gradually increases at its anterior border and, therefore, the endocardial level there becomes elevated. This elevation gradually becomes higher downward, and a portion of cell cords of the anterior division enters the elevation. The cell cords are separated from the remaining cell cords by ever-increasing connective tissue fibers (about 2.3 cm below the aortic leaflets; here, I will again emphasize that the preparation is cut horizontally, i.e. vertically to the septum). The elevated process gradually becomes higher and more round and, consequently, its connection with the septal endocardium gradually becomes poorer until the process is entirely separated from the septum. Thus, the main portion of the anterior division enters a cord which runs very far downward through the ventricular cavity and finally reaches the large anterior papillary muscle, as shown in the subsequent serial sections. The remaining anterior division still runs downward in the subendocardium, although it becomes very slender.

The larger posterior division of the left bundle branch runs vertically downward as a relatively prominent bundle always in the subendocardium and it becomes thicker inferiorly. During its course, no significant twig splits from the bundle. Several small twigs, however, enter the adjacent cardiac musculature (sections No. 46–85). Here, preparation No. IV ended. Preparation No. V serves as a continuation of No. IV. In this preparation, the manner in which the terminal twigs of the left bundle branch spread in all portions of the left ventricle is especially well seen. It would be redundant to repeat all the findings in detail. Instead, I will limit myself to describing only the further course of the anterior division which I have already partly described.

As mentioned above, the anterior division is itself already divided into two groups. The bigger group enters a tendinous fiber-like cord and the smaller still remains in the subendocardium, extending downward with a thickness of only two to three cells through a tendinous cord. The tendinous cord is surrounded by strong connective tissue on its myocardial side and by the endocardium on its outer side. Embedded in the connective tissue mass, the cell cords extend through the tendinous cord to its other end. Here, it is noteworthy that this relatively small tendinous cord possesses thick subendocardial fatty tissue almost throughout its length. The cord, however, is nowhere completely surrounded by fatty tissue. Mostly, fatty tissue surrounds the cord falciformly with its concave surface and a variable portion of the cord is left free from fatty tissue (Fig. 11). The thickness of the cell cords running in the cord is extraordinarily variable. Moreover, there are significant thickness variations even in a single cell cord within a short distance. The number of cells standing side by side and regulating the thickness of a cell cord also varies greatly. For example, as many as 40–45 cells running inside the connective tissue are counted in a cross-sectional surface. Such a thick cell cord never extends for a long distance. Already in the next sections, straight or bent, or seldom Y-formed, connective tissue usually appears in a cell group and divides it into two or three cell groups. In the subsequent sections, each of the cell groups forms an independent cell cord with its own connective tissue sheath. In this way, a cell cord ramifies into two or three cell cords. These cords further ramify or, on the other hand, combine and join each other again into one cord (cf. Fig. 11). Thus, these cell cords always form a long but narrow meshed network in a relatively small connective tissue cord. It can be easily recognized from the above descriptions why the number and size of the cell cords change so markedly even in a small cord and within a short distance. This description is applicable not only for this connective tissue cord, but also for all other similar cords, and also for all subendocardial cell cords, already known as Purkinje fibers.

I will not go into greater detail. Instead, I will describe the further course of the anterior division of the left bundle branch. The connective tissue cord, in which the main portion of the cell cords enter, runs approximately 8 mm through the ventricular cavity downward and branches into two twigs. The bigger twig runs further downward and attaches to the middle portion of the big anterior papillary muscle, radiating its cell cords to all directions in the subendocardium of the papillary muscle, especially down toward the apex of the heart. The other twig of the connective tissue cord is itself shortly divided into two twigs. One of them runs transversely and soon attaches to the anteroinferior portion of the septum. Another runs downward and combines with a twig of connective tissue cord, which will be described soon (cf. Fig. 11).

As already mentioned, the remaining anterior division runs inferiorly in the subendocardium as only two or three cell cords. One of these cell cords enters a small connective tissue cord. This cord leaves the septum and extends through the ventricular cavity to another part of the wall, whilst the remaining two cell cords run further inferiorly in the subendocardium, gradually separating from each other. The single cell cord, entering the above-mentioned connective tissue cord and leaving the septum, branches into many cell cords during its course and forms a narrow meshed network within the small connective tissue cord. The connective tissue cord is divided into two twigs after a short distance. One twig soon attaches to the lower portion of the anterior parietal wall, i.e. between the anterior papillary muscle and the ventricular septum. The other connects with the above-mentioned twig of the connective tissue cord which contains the main mass of the anterior division. This unified connective tissue cord runs further downward and reaches the base of the anterior papillary muscle. From all the attachments of the twigs of the connective tissue cords, Purkinje fibers spread radially in various directions.

So far, I have described only the smaller anterior division of the left bundle branch. This division spread mainly to the anterior papillary muscle, the lower one-third of the anterior half of the ventricular septum, and a portion of the parietal wall between the ventricular septum and the anterior papillary muscle.

I will not describe in such detail the larger posterior division of the left bundle branch, because it spreads principally in a fashion analogous to the anterior division. It sends a special twig of cell cords through a connective tissue cord to the posterior papillary muscle, and the rest of the cell cords spread over the wall of the left ventricle, partly through short or long connective tissue cords extending in the ventricular cavity or partly directly in the subendocardium.

In this way, the main twigs of the left bundle branch spread predominantly to the middle portion of both the papillary muscles and to various portions of the wall, particularly to the lower half of the middle one-third and the upper half of the lower one-third of the left ventricle. From each attachment of the main twigs, many cell cords spread in various directions as the terminal ramifications. These terminal ramifications consist either of one cell cord, or of several cell cords lying side by side or one upon another, and form a (primary) network by connecting with each other. On the other hand, the terminal ramifications in many ways connect or branch and form a widely spreading (secondary) network.

In addition to these highly traceable main twigs, I recognized in various sites in all the sections numerous cell cords or cell cord groups which lay mainly in the subendocardium, often between cardiac muscle bundles. These cell cords are usually sectioned in a crosswise fashion, but not infrequently obliquely or longitudinally. They never connected directly with the left bundle branch in its course mentioned earlier. Furthermore, I frequently observed how a cell cord, branching from a subendocardial cell cord, runs into the cardiac muscle as a straight or usually curved process accompanied by connective tissue fibers and divides again into many twigs. When one single section is observed, the intramuscular cell cords are recognized as cell islands scattered between the ordinary cardiac muscle bundles. When the sections are serially observed, however, the connection between the islands and the subendocardial cell cords is always confirmed. I could not be sure whether those intramuscular cell cords reach the pericardium, although I made numerous preparations through the full thickness of the right parietal wall of this heart. It is possible that the terminal ramifications might very seldom reach the subpericardial connective tissue. Their frequent appearance in the subpericardium, nonetheless, is denied. The cell cords of the terminal ramifications of this system connect with the cardiac muscle fibers in all cardiac muscle layers.

Now, I wanted to establish through serial sections the relationship between the seemingly scattered cell groups in all parts of the ventricular wall and the terminal twigs of the left bundle branch. I was only partly successful, however, because numerous final twigs were divided into too many terminal ramifications, ran in too many directions, and formed nets too complicated to be pursued precisely under a microscope. What I could not be sure of under a microscope, however, was confirmed relatively well with the naked eye in another heart. I will, therefore, describe these macroscopic findings briefly.

Macroscopic finding of the terminal ramifications of the atrioventricular connecting bundle of the sheep heart

It has generally been known since the writings of Purkinje that the fibers coined after his name are very well seen macroscopically in both the right and the left ventricular endocardium in various animal hearts, especially in the sheep heart. About 60 years ago, Purkinje recognized macroscopically these fibers in the sheep endocardium. He studied them precisely and found that they were composed of a number of peculiar large "corns." In the fresh heart, the fibers appear somewhat paler, clearer or more gray than the gray-reddish shining surface of the surroundings. When the fibers are accompanied by yellow–white fatty tissue on both sides, as is often the case, they are recognized especially well. In a heart fixed in Formol-Müller solution and then preserved in alcohol, the fibers look green–gray, whereas the remaining cardiac muscles are stained more brown–gray. In this condition, these fibers are highly visible through the accompanying fatty tissue on both sides. In a heart fixed in Kaiserling solution, the fibers are not well recognizable, because the myocardium is stained red–brown, and the fibers are also stained with almost the same color. In such a heart, the courses of the fibers are only recognized by the accompanying fatty tissue.

In all hearts, these fibers, branching and reunifying, form a large network spreading on the ventricular inner surface. Their meshes are sometimes large and sometimes small, taking various forms. Heßling regarded the larger diameter of the meshes — in other words, the main direction of the fiber courses — as running parallel to the vertical axis of the heart. Obermeier, in contrast, considered the direction to be transverse. It is, however, not easy to decide. From my viewpoint, except for the direction of the fibers around both the large papillary muscles, the fibers in the left ventricle predominantly run parallel to the longitudinal axis of the heart. In the papillary muscles, from the sites of attachment of the connective tissue cords existing in all the sheep hearts, major Purkinje fibers run radially like the roots of a tree and connect with the neighboring parts of the ventricular wall. Also, from the anterior papillary muscle, the fibers run radially in all directions in the parietal wall of the right ventricle. In the right surface of the ventricular septum, however, the direction of the fibers is predominantly parallel to the anterior line of the transition from the septum to the parietal wall.

These Purkinje fibers can be seen in all parts of the walls both in the right and left ventricles. In contrast to Obermeier's viewpoint, however, there is a certain difference regarding the number and the thickness of the fibers, depending on their locations in the ventricle. I recognized in all the sheep hearts that the fibers were most frequently and clearly seen in the lower two-thirds of both the ventricles, especially around the papillary muscles. On the other hand, the fibers are seldom and unclearly seen in the upper one-third of both the ventricles, and only sparsely seen near the semilunar and the atrioventricular valves. Each of the fibers lies on the relatively smooth ventricular muscular surface, and is covered by the endocardium. The endocardial level at the place where Purkinje fibers run is often somewhat more elevated than the surroundings. These endocardial elevations are especially marked arround the papillary muscles. At uneven places where big trabeculations develop, or the papillary muscles originate, or at the transition from the septum to the parietal wall, the fibers do not always simply run on the muscular surface but take a short cut in a lifted endocardial fold. At the place where recesses are deeper, the fibers run in the form of a small, short, bridgelike connective tissue cord (so called false tendinous fiber). These short bridges are frequently seen between each trabeculation in both the ventricles, especially at the anterior and posterior transitions from the septum to the parietal wall of the right ventricle, at the lower one-third of the left ventricle, and between each papillary muscle and the adjacent ventricular wall.

Not infrequently, there are longer and fine tendinous fiber-like cords extending from one point to another through the ventricular cavity. The cords often extend from the anterior papillary muscle of the right ventricle or its neighboring area to the posterior papillary muscle or to the ventricular septum. *All these cords in both of the inner ventricular walls are exclusively for the terminal ramifications of the atrioventricular connecting bundle.* (Of course, these cords are not true tendinous fibers attaching to the valve leaflets.)

When you consider that both the bundle branches of the atrioventricular connecting bundle give forth no subendocardial or intramuscular twigs during their upper courses, as demonstrated microscopically in preparation No. 155, and further that the right bundle branch first spreads at the anterior papillary muscle, and the left bundle branch first spreads at the anterior and posterior papillary muscles and at various parts of the wall between the two papillary muscles, then the subendocardial networks in these areas described macroscopically must be identical to those subendocardial terminal ramifications of both the bundle branches described microscopically.

Consequently, the evidence is that the left as well as the right bundle branch is connected with the networks which spread subendocardially on the ventricular inner surfaces, and that all the subendocardial networks are nothing but the terminal ramifications of the left as well as the right bundle branch. Especially interesting is that the terminal ramifications do not run downward from the ventricular base, as usually considered, but spread inversely from the vicinity of the apex of the heart, especially from the papillary muscles, in all directions (i.e. inversely toward the ventricular base as well as toward the apex of the heart). From these subendocardial networks, numerous twigs go into the muscle layers and connect with cardiac muscle fibers at various sites. This connection is numerously recognized in the subendocardial muscle layer.

I cannot say with certainty whether there is any connection between the terminal ramifications of the left and the right bundle branch. This probability must be very small. If such connections exist, the connection should be insignificant, because, as far as I had examined, there were no such connections between the main branches of both the bundles.

Finally, the fact should be emphasized that nerve bundles constantly accompany the atrioventricular connecting bundle of heart No. 155. Namely, there are several small nerve bundles coming through the atrial septum and entering the atrial segment of the atrioventricular connecting bundle which consists of the muscular networks of thin fibers. The nerve bundles extend anteroinferiorly to the ventricular septum, together with the bundle. From the dividing portion of the bundle, a part of the nerve bundles goes a long distance downward along with the left bundle branch, and another part along with the right bundle branch. In the right bundle branch, I easily followed the accompanying nerve bundle up to the papillary muscle. I also recognized the nerve bundles well up to the anterior and posterior divisions of the left bundle branch. These nerves do not always run as a closed bundle, but divide into two or three small bundles between the cell cords and then reunify, thus forming a long stretched network. I cannot say whether these nerve fibers connect with each cell of the cell cords, because I did not perform any special nerve staining.

(2) *No. 160. The sheep heart**

The situation of the atrioventricular connecting bundle was generally the same as that described for heart No. 155, although there were small

---

*Photographs of the sheep heart together with a tracing on which the course of the connecting bundle is drawn in red are given in Plate III, Fig. 2, and Plate IV, Fig. 1.

differences. I describe this heart briefly, therefore, comparing it with heart No. 155.

When observed from the left, at the height of the lowest attachment of the noncoronary aortic leaflet, and when observed from the right, starting about 5 mm beneath the lower margin of the oval fossa, i.e. from the anteroinferior portion of the coronary sinus and stretching forwardly to the inferoposterior portion of the membranous septum, the typical entirely irregularly knitted network is seen for the first time to be consisting of striated thin muscle fibers. The network lies on the right half of the atrial septum, about 2 mm apart from the right endocardium, and nestles close on the atrioventricular fibrocartilaginous septum. The posteroanterior longitudinal axis is almost horizontal, bending slightly downward at its anterior tip. The largest horizontal size is about 4×1.2 mm. Its form seems to be that of a long irregular ellipsoid. Posteriorly, to the right and above, it connects with the seemingly ordinary cardiac muscle fibers, which peculiarly also connect with each other and form a widely meshed network. A part of these muscle fibers goes through extensive fatty tissue occupying the middle of the atrial septum up to a muscle group on the left half of the atrial septum and connects with the muscle group. The remaining part of the muscle fibers extends upward, rightward and posteriorly and connects at various sites with the ordinary atrial muscle fibers running relatively parallel to each other. The formation of a network of these seemingly ordinary muscle fibers was not so clear as such in heart No. 155. Nevertheless, I could recognize it relatively well.

When the network of small fibers is traced forward, just at the entrance of the canal penetrating from the right anterior to the left posterior, its sudden transition to a network of irregularly formed and striated large cells, as described for heart No. 155, is also seen in this heart. This network of large cells first extends anteroinferiorly, then almost vertically downward. Within a short distance, the network divides into the two bundle branches and the bundle branches gradually separate from each other.

The right bundle branch first runs downward and somewhat forward, then forward and somewhat downward. Passing by the base of a tendinous fiber belonging to the septal leaflet of the tricuspid valve, it runs almost vertically downward. Then, after running about 1.7 cm, it enters a big, about 1.5-cm-long muscular trabeculation and, through this muscle bridge, directly extends to the anterior papillary muscle flatly seated on the parietal wall. The right bundle branch finally spreads in all directions. In this heart, the right bundle branch gives forth no subendocardial twigs during its course, never reaching the right endocardium and running in the cardiac musculature at least 1 mm apart from the endocardium. On the other hand, in heart No. 155, the right bundle branch runs for a short extent in the subendocardium, and in the hearts of human and dog, it mostly runs in the subendocardium.

In contrast to all the other hearts I have examined thus far, the left bundle branch is much smaller than the right in this case. Beneath the right half of the noncoronary aortic leaflet, it reaches the left subendocardial connective tissue and runs vertically downward. After running about 1.8 cm, its major portion enters a connective tissue cord about 1 mm thick, whereas the minor portion runs further downward in the subendocardium. The connective tissue cord soon divides into two twigs which run further for about 1.3 and 1.2 cm and attach to the anterior and posterior papillary muscles, respectively. From each of these two twigs, several further twigs arise which, during their downward courses, form several meshes by either connecting or dividing among themselves. Several meshes attach to the lower portion of both the papillary muscles, while the remaining meshes reach various parts of the wall at the lower one-third of the ventricle. From all these attachments, subendocardial terminal ramifications spread to all portions of the inner surface of the wall, and also extend upward to the ventricular base.

(e) *Calf heart*

(1) *No. 158. The calf heart*

In this heart, the important part of the ventricular septum was studied in serial sections and the remaining part was examined macroscopically. In preparation No. I, the septum including the atrioventricular fibrocartilaginous septum was sectioned in series horizontally, parallel to the closing edge of the noncoronary and the right coronary aortic leaflet, approximately to the same extent as preparation No. I of the sheep heart (No. 155). Preparations No. III and No. II are the downward continuation of preparation No. I.

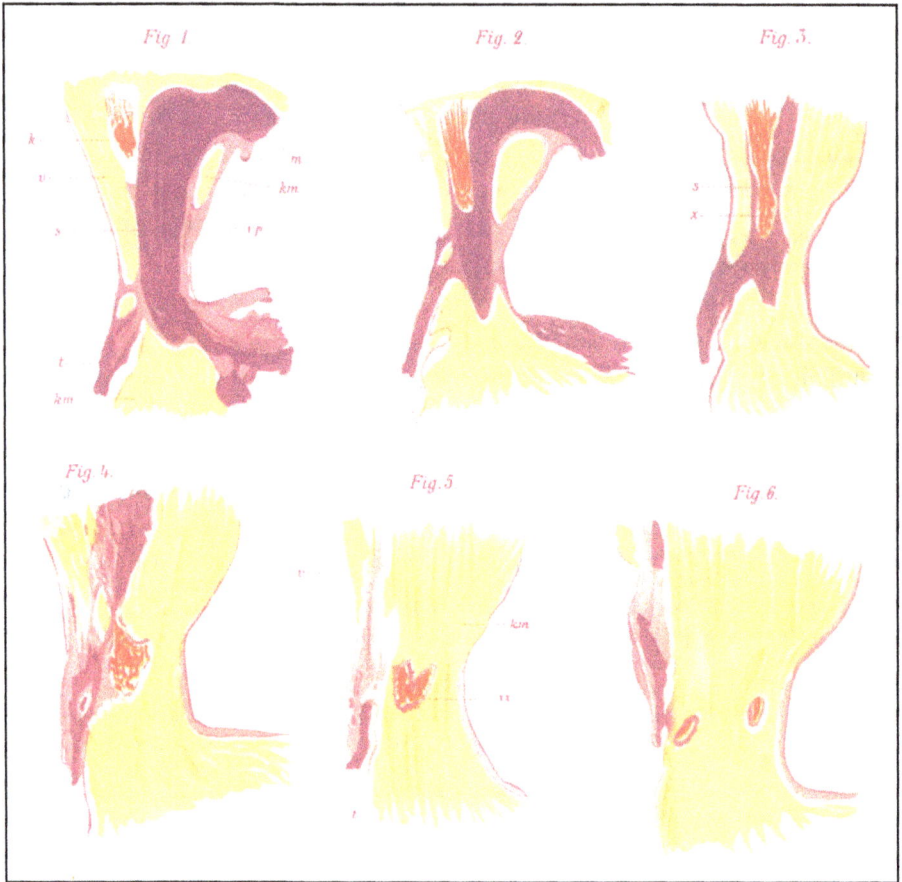

Calf heart No. 158

v, *k*, *s*, *m*, *z*, *km*, *vp*, *l* and *r* are the same as for sheep heart No. 155

x = the connecting bundle penetrates the atrioventricular fibrocartilaginous septum, entering the ventricular septum

xx = the ventricular bundle of the connecting system is divided into two bundle branches

(continued on next page)

(*continued from previous page*)

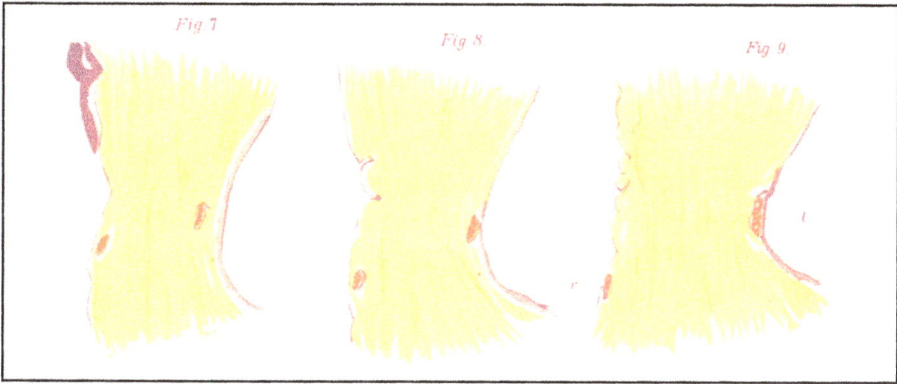

Preparation No. III contains the continuation of the left bundle branch, whilst preparation No. II carries the continuation of the right bundle branch. The descriptions of the sheep heart No. 155 can be compared.

Through examination of preparation No. I, for the first time in section No. 28, a small peculiarly arranged muscle group (*k*) is seen. In the next two sections, it enlarges very rapidly to become a considerable mass. These muscle fibers are very small and look quite different from the ordinary atrial muscle fibers. The muscle fibers have longitudinal and transverse striations. The fiber width is not as regular as the ordinary atrial muscle fibers. The irregularity in width is observed not only among the fibers, but also within a single fiber. The fibers connect with each other and form an irregular network which looks quite different from the netlike formation of the ordinary cardiac muscle fibers. The knots of the net are usually wide and flat and contain one or more nuclei which partly lie in a clear halo. The muscle fibrils usually run in highly intricate patterns in the knot and radiate into the other fibers starting from the knot. Each of the fibers of this muscle group does not run close and parallel to each other, but rather extends in various directions and connects with others at an obtuse angle. A complicated network is therefore formed, and its meshes are sometimes big and sometimes small, with various shapes. Here, these meshes are filled with loose connective tissue fibers and fatty tissue.

The highest point of this peculiar netlike structure lies at the height of the lowest attachment of the noncoronary aortic leaflet (*ap*) when observed from the left, and approximately 4–5 mm above the middle portion of the attachment of the septal leaflet of the tricuspid valve (*t*) when observed from the right. The network structure nestles to the right side of the origin of the aorta which consists of cartilaginous tissue, forming a part of the atrioventricular fibrocartilaginous septum, and faces the lowest attachment of the noncoronary aortic leaflet. From the right, its greater part is separated from the ordinary atrial musculature (*v*) by thick connective tissue. Here and there, the thick connective tissue is interrupted and the peculiar muscle fibers occasionally connect with the ordinary atrial muscle fibers at the sites of interruption. At the posterior extent of the net, the connective tissue is not well developed and numerous muscle fibers of the network connect with the atrial muscle fibers, extending here not as compact and parallel ordinary atrial muscle bundles but as loose muscle groups in various directions, especially toward the posterior. The atrial muscle fibers running divergently in a peculiar fashion in various directions very often connect with each other, usually by a relatively long connecting arm, and here form a widely meshed network. This network, however, is not as prominent as that of the sheep heart No. 155. Also, the atrial muscle fibers forming the net connect with the ordinary atrial muscles lying in various sites as well as in relatively remote sites of the atrial septum. Not only between the muscle fibers of the first-mentioned small fiber network, but also between those of the last-mentioned atrial fiber net, there is abundant connective tissue, and fatty tissue is sporadically observed. In addition, several strikingly large nerve bundles appear here (Fig. I = section No. 29).

In the sections which follow (No. 31–34), the plexus of small fibers gradually enlarges posteriorly. The plexus always nestles close to the right of the fibrocartilaginous septum (in this description, the heart is upright with the base upward and the apex downward, the ventricular septum being placed anteroposteriorly in the sagittal direction; the naming of the sites may be different when the heart is in its natural position) and, from the right, the plexus is sharply demarcated from the ordinary atrial muscle fibers by connective tissue, i.e. the right posterior continuation of the atrioventricular fibrocartilaginous septum. Only at its posterior extent do the muscle fibers of the network still connect with the atrial muscle fibers.

This connection, however, gradually becomes sparse, because more fatty tissue, numerous large nerve bundles and loose connective tissue appear here. Consequently, there exists only a small amount of the atrial muscle fibers (Fig. 2 = section No. 34).

From section No. 35, the front tip of the small fiber network gradually elongates anteriorly and connects with another network, the fibers of which have an entirely different property. At a weak magnification, each fiber of this new network looks generally much thicker than that of the small fiber network. These thick fibers branch and connect with each other, forming a network. In general, the arrangement of this fiber network looks totally analogous to that of the small fiber network. The only difference is that the fibers are much thicker and the meshes much wider. When the thick fibers are observed at a stronger magnification, an entirely different arrangement is recognized. Namely, the fibers consist of large, differently shaped and mostly polyhedral cells having one or two, or seldom three, nuclei usually lying in a relatively large clear halo. By connecting serially with each other, such large cells form a fiber. In a cross section, two to four cells stand close side by side. These cell groups also form a fiber by connecting with each other. The thickness of these fibers is markedly different. Usually, the fibers do not run straight but curve irregularly and connect with others at an obtuse angle. In this way, a very irregular network is made. The borders of the cells can usually be well seen. The border is here and there difficult to be recognized, so that the cells appear to be a long fiber, in which there are nuclei in several places. At the knots of the network, many polyhedral cells can often be observed lying pressed on each other. These cells have numerous cross-striated fibrils or fibril bundles, mostly running in various directions. The fibrils at the peripheral portion of the cells are especially well seen. Thus, the fibrils seem to continue to run from one cell to another. Therefore, longitudinal and cross striations are recognized not only in each cell but also in the fibers composed of these cells. Moreover, these cells often appear homogenous and exhibit fine granules only at the periphery. The fine granules, however, are nothing but fibrils or small fibril bundles sectioned crosswise. At the knot of the network, the fibrils run often in a complicated arrangement and without interruption enter cell cords which depart from the knot. At the transition from the network of large cells to that of small fibers, the fibrils also run without interruption from one cell to another.

In the subsequent sections, the network of small fibers lying posteriorly becomes more extensive and, in section No. 38, attains its greatest horizontal cross diameter (about 2.3 mm). The network, however, gradually reduces its size from the posterior due to appearance of increasing amounts of fatty tissue, connective tissue and abundant nerve bundles. Only the right posterior corner of the network is connected with the atrial musculature. From the left, the network is bordered by the origin of the aorta, i.e. by part of the fibrocartilaginous septum. From the right, it is bordered by the above-mentioned connective tissue. The distance between the network of small fibers and the right-side endocardium of the atrial septum is about 1 mm. Anteriorly, it connects directly with the network of large cells. It does not extend any more anteriorly. From section No. 39, the network of small fibers becomes rapidly smaller and disappears in section No. 45. The network is replaced by connective tissue, fatty tissue and large nerve bundles.

The network of large fibers gradually lengthens anteriorly and takes a conical form. It lies close to the atrioventricular fibrocartilaginous septum, first inserting its conical anterior tip between the cartilage and the thick connective tissue attaching to the cartilage, and then penetrating the fibro-cartilaginous tissue. Finally, in section No. 40, it perforates the cartilage. In this case, when seen from the left ventricle, the site of perforation is about 1.2 mm below the lowest attachment of the noncoronary aortic leaflet, and it is posterior to the right half of the leaflet. The site is separated from the left endocardium by the ventricular musculature (*km*) of about 2.5 mm thickness. When seen from the right, the site is about 2–3 mm above the anterior half of the attachment of the septal leaflet of the tricuspid valve, and about 1.5 mm from the right-side endocardium. The horizontal width of the perforating canal is about 0.8 mm at its narrowest. The nerve bundles in the meshes of the network of small fibers decompose into numerous small bundles or individual nerve fibers, spread all over the meshes of the network of large cells and accompany the network toward the venticular septum (Fig. 3 = section No. 40).

From section No. 41, the network of large cells not only runs anteriorly but also widens its size very rapidly. At the tip of the bundle, both the knots of the network and the individual cell cords are especially well developed. The knots are very large discs composed of many cells. In sections No. 43 and No. 44, the posterior portion of the network of large cells is surrounded by connective tissue and is separated from the network of small fibers. The network of small fibers, still seen here as a modest mass as stated above, rapidly disappears in the next two to three sections. At this area, the ventricular portion of the large cell bundle does not yet lie as a whole in the ventricular muscle but is separated from the ventricular musculature (*km*) left anteriorly by the partly hyaline and partly fibrous cartilage of the origin of the aortia, i.e. a part below the right half of the attachment of the noncoronary aortic leaflet and also of a part of the atrioventricular fibrocartilaginous septum (*s*). On the other hand, its right side is bordered in most of its extension by a part of the atrioventricular fibrocartilaginous septum. Only at its right posterior portion does it lie close to the ventricular musculature. In the following sections, the rest of the origin of the aorta rapidly disappears, and in section No. 45, the greater part of the large cell bundle is already surrounded by the ventricular musculature (*km*) except for its right side, where the bundle is bordered by a loose but thick connective tissue forming the base of the septal leaflet of the tricuspid valve (*t*) and also belonging to the atrioventricular fibrocartilaginous septum (Fig. 4 = section No. 45).

Here, in a horizontal plane, the large cell bundle has the shape of a round anisoceles triangle, the shortest side of which is about 1.7 mm and the longest about 2.5 mm. The bundle is surrounded by a connective tissue sheath and has four to five relatively large nerve bundles at its periphery. The meshes of the bundle are filled with loose connective tissue fibers, numerous small nerve bundles or nerve fibers and small blood vessels. Now, this network extends no longer forward but vertically downward. The distance from the bundle to both the right and the left endocardium is about the same. In section No. 49, the network is divided into two bundle branches, the right and the left, which gradually separate from each other in the subsequent sections. In the beginning, the right bundle branch is somewhat thicker than the left. Both the bundle branches are sharply separated from the adjacent ventricular musculature by a connective tissue sheath (Fig. 5 = section No. 49).

The left bundle branch (*l*) runs almost vertically downward and, at the same time, gradually moves left anteriorly. It becomes gradually somewhat smaller and, from section No. 70, again somewhat larger. In section No. 81, it reaches the left subendocardial thick connective tissue, i.e. about 7 mm below the lowest attachment of the noncoronary aortic leaflet and approximately on the vertical line running inferiorly between the right coronary and noncoronary aortic leaflets (Figs. 6, 7 and 8 = sections No. 60, 71 and 83). Until this point, it is always surrounded by a connective tissue sheath and is sharply separated from the adjacent ventricular musculature. The gaps between individual large cell cords, namely the network meshes, are relatively wide and highly irregular. In the meshes of the network, there are connective tissue fibers, a number of small blood vessels or capillaries, and especially rich nerve bundles or nerve fibers. The individual cell cords are sectioned differently. The cords run not always parallel to the direction of the bundle, but in various directions, and always form a net by combining with each other.

After reaching the subendocardium, the left bundle branch runs further vertically downward. The number of cell cords gradually increases and, by joining each other, scattered nerve fibers coalesce into several relatively large bundles, which accompany the left bundle branch further downward. The nerve bundles seem to run a twisted course, because they are sectioned sometimes crosswise, sometimes obliquely and sometimes longitudinally. They form a nerve plexus inside the left bundle branch by combining and dividing with each other. Here, the individual cell cords extend downward running mostly parallel to each other. The greater part of the cords, therefore, are sectioned crosswise. A few connecting cell cords between the parallel cell cords are cut obliquely. The crosswise sections of the cell cords demonstrate mostly three to seven palely stained large cells lying close side by side. At the periphery of the cells, and not infrequently at their center, there are numerous granules of various sizes. There are often chances to observe, especially in the cells sectioned obliquely or longitudinally, that the cells have cross-striated fibrils and that the above-mentioned granules are nothing but cross sections of the fibrils. When they are observed carefully, it is found that the larger granules are composed of several finer fibrils. On the other hand, smaller granules are composed of less or only one fibril. The individual cells of various shapes have one or two beautiful, spherical or longish oval nuclei usually lying one after another in the longitudinal direction of the cell cords. In this subendocardium, the individual cell cords already demonstrate typical characteristics of the well-known Purkinje fibers in all respects (Fig. 9 = section No. 96).

In this case, it is especially noteworthy that some ganglion cells were found in one of the nerve bundles in section No. 106. The site is about 1.2 cm below the aortic valvar leaflet. The numerous nerve bundles run in close connection with the connecting bundle from the atrial segment, i.e. the small fiber network, up to here. I could not recognize any ganglion cells so far during this long distance. Unexpectedly, this happened now for the first time.

This serial preparation ended here at section No. 112. I will follow further continuation of the left bundle branch in another preparation No. III, made for this purpose.

In the new sections, the direct continuation of the left bundle branch can be seen lying in the subendocardium and having a rounded triangular form. One side of the triangle lies on thick and strong subendocardial connective tissue. The tip opposing this side of the triangle wedges into the adjacent ordinary cardiac muscle, from which the tip is separated by connective tissue. The thickness of the left bundle branch is about 1 mm at this site, about 1.3 cm below the aortic leaflet. In the following sections, the left bundle branch gradually becomes smaller and the number of the cell cords slightly decreases. On average, the individual cell cords are small in size and have mostly three to six, seldom more, cells in their cross sections. Further down, the left bundle branch gradually widens anteriorly in the subendocardium. The thickness, on the other hand, reduces and several cell cords, especially at the anterior portion of the left bundle branch, run obliquely or partly horizontally. (In section No. 34, the width of the bundle is about 2.8 mm and the thickness is only 0.3 mm at the site about 2 cm below the aortic leaflets.) Until here, although rare, ganglion cells are also observed scattered in the accompanying nerve bundles. In addition, the left bundle branch is always accompanied by numerous small blood vessels and capillaries. The bundle branch is further accompanied by two relatively large vessels which appear from the septum at a height about 5 mm below the aortic valvar leaflets. These enter the left bundle branch and run down always with the bundle branch.

In the following sections, the subendocardial width of the left bundle branch gradually becomes greater. It is eventually divided into two groups: the anterior, smaller division and the posterior, larger division. At the same time, the numerous nerve bundles also divide into two groups and accompany the divisions of the cell cords. The cell cords of the anterior division become a bundle by joining together and the bundle gradually enters an about 1.2-mm-thick connective tissue cord which emerges from the septum about 2.8 cm below the aortic leaflets and extends through the ventricular cavity to the anterior papillary muscle. The number of the cell cords of this group is approximately eight to ten at the entrance to the connective tissue cord. The size of each cell cord, however, is relatively large. The cell cords contain not infrequently over 20 cells in cross section. The individual cell cords are provided with their own connective tissue sheaths. The cell cords often divide into two, sometimes three, cell cords or connect with other during their courses. In this way, a long stretched net is formed inside the connective tissue cord.

The larger posterior division is about 2 mm wide but very thin. Further down, it becomes slender as its anterior portion reduces. Accordingly, the posterior division is gradually distanced from the anterior. The individual cell cords of the posterior division run vertically downward and become, on average, much thicker than before. Like the anterior division, most of the cell cords, arranged as a bundle, enter a connective tissue cord about 3 cm below the aortic leaflets and leave the muscular layer of the septum. The remaining small number of cell cords continue further to take their course in the subendocardium.

In this calf heart, extraordinarily numerous nerve bundles always accompany the left bundle branch. Some of them have already left the left bundle branch and run in other directions either in the subendocardium or in the myocardium. In the left bundle branch, however, there still remain many nerve bundles which enter the connective tissue cords together with the twigs of the left bundle branch. I cannot say with absolute certainty whether these nerve bundles have any close relationships with the cells of the connecting bundle. I tend to accept, nonetheless, that the two elements are connected with each other, because they always run closely arranged as stated above.

In its long course up to now, the left bundle branch was totally separated from the adjacent musculature by connective tissue. Only in the last sections did I see several insignificant cell cords connected to the adjacent ordinary muscle fibers of the septum.

This serial preparation No. III ended here at section No. 74. In this case, I did not make any further serial sections of the left ventricle. Therefore, I will describe macroscopically the course of the left bundle branch in the same heart preserved in alcohol.*

The anterior division of the left bundle branch enters a connective tissue cord about 1.2 mm thick and 1.8 cm long which runs obliquely through the ventricular cavity and is divided into three twigs at its end, attaching to the middle portion of the large anterior papillary muscle. When the sites of attachment of each twig to the papillary muscle are observed precisely, it is clearly seen that fine final twigs spread radially in the subendocardium in all directions from the sites of attachment. Sometimes as thin and sometimes as wide fibers, the twigs form a very tight and irregular network by connecting and branching with each other. The network is especially well seen inferiorly, i.e. toward the apex of the heart. It also runs from the surface of the papillary muscle to the adjacent wall. Moreover, this anterior connective tissue cord gives forth a twig in its upper portion. While running downward, the twig is divided into three twigs attaching to various sites of the septum.

The larger posterior division of the left bundle branch is divided into two groups, as mentioned above. The smaller one runs further vertically downward in the subendocardium and is recognized macroscopically to run almost to the apex of the heart. On the other hand, the larger one, as a closed bundle, enters a connective tissue cord and extends through the ventricular cavity to the middle portion of the large posterior papillary muscle. At its attachment, this posterior larger group is suddenly divided into numerous twigs which spread radially from here in all directions in the subendocardium over the entire surface of the papillary muscle, especially downward to the apex of the heart, forming a net. Terminal ramifications also extend from the papillary muscle to various adjacent sites on the ventricular wall. This posterior connective tissue cord, about 1.2 cm long, is in symmetric relationship with the anterior cord described earlier. The posterior cord gives forth a short twig from its upper portion. The twig immediately attaches to the adjacent wall and its cell cords spread

---

*The course of the connecting bundle of a bovine heart is given in the photographs with attached tracings in Plate IV, Fig. 2, and Plate V, Figs. 1 and 2.

vertically in the subendocardium running upward to the ventricular base. This short twig sends another long thin twig which, while running downward, again gives forth three short smaller twigs, toward various posterior wall sites, and finally attaches to the base of the posterior papillary muscle.

Briefly summarized in this case, the left bundle branch for the first time gives rise to the subendocardial terminal ramifications at the middle portion of both the papillary muscles and at various wall sites of the lower half of the middle and the upper half of the lower one-third of the left ventricle. The ramifications form a wide net and spread to all wall portions, i.e. to the apex and also to the base of the ventricle.

At the beginning (from section No. 49 of preparation No. I), the right bundle branch runs almost vertically downward, somewhat anteriorly and toward the right-side endocardium of the septum. The right bundle branch rapidly separates from the left. The bundle is thicker than that of the left bundle branch at the beginning, but becomes gradually smaller as it extends downward. The bundle has numerous nerve fiber bundles, sometimes large and sometimes small. The nerve bundles occupy proportionally larger space, so that the large cell cords still forming here a widely meshed net appear to lie scattered between them. In addition, numerous small blood vessels or capillaries are seen between the cell cords or connective tissue fibers. The individual cell cords are mostly sectioned here more or less longitudinally. The width of the cell cord varies, because the cell cords are composed of many, or sometimes a few, cells arranged horizontally. Even in a cell cord, the difference in width occurs so prominently that the cell cord appears to be very irregular, sometimes thin and sometimes thick. On average, cell cords have three to five cells in cross section. The cords are relatively small but the number of the cell cords is relatively large. All the cell cords appear to have their own connective tissue sheaths. They are further surrounded by a common connective tissue sheath and are separated from the adjacent musculature. In section No. 56, the right bundle branch is as large as the left, but the number of cell cords is smaller in the right, and both the bundle branches run in an almost symmetric position in the septum at approximately the same distance from both the endocardiums (for example, about 0.6 mm in section No. 56). From here, the right bundle branch runs somewhat forward and each of the cell cords appears to become gradually larger. Its connective tissue sheath becomes more distinct. In section No. 65, the (horizontal) sectional form of the right bundle branch is a beautiful blunt spindle. In the following sections, it becomes longer and, at the same time, moves gradually forward. In section No. 70, the right bundle branch is separated from the right-side endocardium only by a thin muscle layer. Downward, the cell cords are stained gradually more transparently and show typical characteristics of the well-known Purkinje fibers. Spaces between the individual cell cords — in other words, net meshes — are entirely filled with nerve bundles, so that there remain almost no gaps in the bundle branch. Here, the net meshes are no longer so wide and irregular as they are at the beginning of the right bundle branch, but mostly narrow and spindly, extending in the same direction as the course of the bundle branch. In this condition, the right bundle branch runs further downward. The number of cell cords decreases and each of the cords becomes thicker. The size of the horizontal section of the right bundle branch is about 0.8×2.0 mm in section No. 53, about 0.5×1.3 mm in section No. 65, and about 0.1×1.1 mm in section No. 110, respectively. The size becomes constantly smaller thereafter when traced downward.

This preparation No. I ended with section No. 112. Preparation No. II is its direct continuation. This contains the continuation of the right bundle branch.

In this serial preparation, the continuation of the right bundle branch is again well recognized. It gradually runs anteroinferiorly. Now, a relatively large blood vessel appears from the upper inner portion of the septum and runs almost vertically downward and somewhat rightward toward the right-side endocardium, i.e. in the course of the right bundle branch. After joining with the blood vessel, the right bundle branch suddenly bends, runs downward, closely related with the vessel, and then enters a muscular trabeculation. Here, this trabeculation leaves the septum (about 1 cm beneath the supraventricular crest) and extends through the ventricular cavity to the base of the anterior papillary muscle nestling flat on the parietal wall. In this case, covered with the endocardium, the trabeculation was about 3 mm thick and 1 cm long. It was mainly composed of the ordinary cardiac musculature.

In this serial preparation No. II, the right bundle branch again becomes gradually larger. The number of cell cords gradually decreases. The size of the individual cell cords, however, becomes larger on average, while more cells appear in the cross-sectional surface here than at the upper portion. During the course of the right bundle branch, the individual cell cords with a connective tissue sheath are divided in acute angles or connect with other cords and still form a long stretched net. This net is closely related with the nerve net accompanying the right bundle branch. In this way, the right bundle branch is composed of the two kinds of nets and is surrounded by a common connective tissue sheath, sharply separated from the adjacent cardiac musculature. Before entering the muscular trabeculation, the right bundle branch never reaches the right-side endocardium. It always runs in the cardiac musculature, at least 0.5 or 1.5 mm apart from the endocardium in its entire course, giving forth neither subendocardial nor intramyocardial twigs.

After entering the muscular trabeculation, the number of cell cords rapidly decreases. The right bundle branch, therefore, becomes smaller. It does not run at the central axis but reaches here the endocardium, extending to the other end of the trabeculation accompanied by the nerve bundles and the blood vessel.

Although extraordinarily manifold in terms of the size and figure, the individual cells are usually large and polyhedral, looking homogeneous and usually possessing one or two beautiful spherical or oval nuclei. In addition, they have numerous fine cross-striated fibrils, or granulations, as described for the left bundle branch.

The further course of the right bundle branch will be followed macroscopically. The muscular trabeculation mentioned above does not directly attach to the anterior papillary muscle in this case, but to the parietal wall lateral to the papillary muscle. From the attachment of the trabeculation, many large final twigs spread in various directions. Such final twigs are large at their initial portion and significantly elevated above the usual level of the endocardium, so that the muscular trabeculation is comparable to a tree trunk firmly cling to rocky ground of less soil with its naked roots. The macroscopically thickest final twig first runs posterosuperiorly, reaches the base of the anterior papillary muscle, and gives forth a thick twig to the papillary muscle. On the other hand, the remaining twigs bend upward, run toward the supraventricular crest and are gradually divided into many barely recognizable twigs. Taking a fan shape along the parietal wall, they spread in the subendocardium toward the tricuspid orifice and the pulmonary infundibulum. The second twig runs posteroinferiorly and is soon divided into many small twigs. They spread from the base of the anterior papillary muscle to the apex of the heart. Moreover, many other final twigs spread anteriorly or inferiorly. *Terminal ramifications of all the final twigs repeatedly connect or ramify with each other and form an interrelated network which is visible everywhere in the right ventricle, especially well at its lower two-thirds.*

The inner surface of the ventricles of this calf heart was relatively smooth. Where there is a deep groove between the trabeculations, or where the parietal wall connects to the septum, short tendinous fiber-like cords bridging the grooves were often seen. They are nothing but the terminal ramifications of the connecting system as demonstrated in the sheep hearts.

When the parts of the wall other than the course of either of the bundle branches are observed, numerous cell cords are seen running in the subendocardium or in the intramyocardium, with numerous connections between the cell cords and the ordinary muscle fibers. As a whole, however, these findings are similar to those on the sheep heart No. 155. Precise description, therefore, is not made here. Only one small difference will be emphasized. In the calf heart, intramyocardial terminal ramifications frequently spread in a flat form between the ordinary cardiac muscle fibers. In this condition, without having an apparently visible connective tissue sheath, the terminal ramifications gradually connected with the cardiac muscle fibers. When observed at weak magnification, a broader, paler and irregular spot exists without a special border between the ordinary cardiac muscle fibers. In the sheep heart, I could never confirm this phenomenon, but the connection between the two muscle elements took place mostly by means of a long narrow cell cord surrounded by a connective tissue sheath up to the site of connection.

Finally, I would like to add one thing. As mentioned before, in this calf heart extraordinarily numerous nerve bundles ran very close together with the muscular atrioventricular connecting bundle and, moreover, scattered ganglion cells appeared in the left bundle branch. I tried to find out the origin of the nerve bundles because, in the descriptions of various books and journals, there has been no consistent view on the fine distribution of cardiac nerves in mammalian animals.

For this purpose, from this calf heart still preserved in alcohol, I cut out two additional pieces of the atrial septum with the posterior atrial wall and serially sectioned them. One preparation is the direct posterior continuation of preparation No. I. This comprises the posteroinferior portion of the atrial septum with the coronary sinus and the part of the atrial wall to which the septum attaches. Therefore, this contains part of the posterior sagittal groove and part of the atrioventricular groove. The other preparation is also the direct continuation of preparation No. I and the superior continuation of the preparation mentioned above. This preparation contains part of the atrial septum with the oval foramen and part of the posterior atrial wall with the upper portion of the posterior sagittal groove.

In these two preparations, numerous nerve bundles with many conspicuous large ganglion cell groups were noticed, especially in the subpericardium around the two grooves. The nerve bundles appeared to be related together. Some penetrated through the muscular and fatty tissue of the posterior atrial wall into the atrial septum and extended anteriorly. The nerve bundles always had ganglion cells which scattered here and there or gathered in a small pile. The nerve bundles mostly ran very wavily, and not infrequently made branchings or connections. Exact tracing, therefore, was very difficult. Besides, the situation in which these three preparations were made independently of each other made it very difficult for me to summarize the findings on the course of the nerve bundles. For these reasons, I cannot say with certainty from where the nerve bundles accompanying the muscular connecting bundle originate. Nevertheless, I think that the nerve bundles — or at least part of them — enter along the atrial septum from the posterior, and that these nerve bundles are connected with the nerve bundles with many ganglion cells mentioned above at the posterior atrial septum. This assumption will be confirmed through further studies.

I further examined two bovine hearts macroscopically. Purkinje fibers are very clearly recognized in the fresh hearts. Although there are small differences in the manner of distribution of the connecting bundle in each heart, it is as a whole similar to that of the calf heart. I do not think that further detailed descriptions are necessary.

II. Histology of the Atrioventricular Connecting System

As I have already emphasized, the muscular system does not show the same features in regard to cellular characteristics and arrangements throughout its extent even in a heart. This interrelated system, extending without interruption to the terminal ramifications, can be histologically divided into many portions. Furthermore, the system demonstrates more or less distinct histological differences in the various animal species examined, so that the terminal ramifications of the system in the human, for example, are substantially different from those seen in the sheep. For these reasons, I will describe the findings for each of the species I examined.

(a) *Sheep heart*

In the sheep heart, the system is divided into two segments from the viewpoint of histological characteristics, namely the atrial and the ventricular segment. The two segments show fundamentally different histological characteristics.

1. *The atrial segment of the connecting bundle*

I have already precisely described the position and form of the bundle of the atrial segment. For simplicity I named it a network of small fibers. When this segment is examined more precisely, it is again seen to be divided into two portions in regard to the arrangement of its constituent bundles, i.e. into the extraordinarily complicated network forming the greater part of the atrial segment and the relatively parallel fibers originating from the right and posterior extent of the network and extending toward the posterior.

Not only is each fiber of the network very thin, but its breadth varies greatly. Here and there, even one muscular fiber shows thicker or thinner parts, so that it never shows equal breadth throughout its length. Fibrils are developed relatively sparsely in these thin muscle fibers compared with those in the ordinary cardiac muscle fibers. The arrangement of the fibrils is very irregular. The fibrils, looking like fine granules of various sizes in cross-sectioned muscle fibers, sometimes scatter all over the sectional

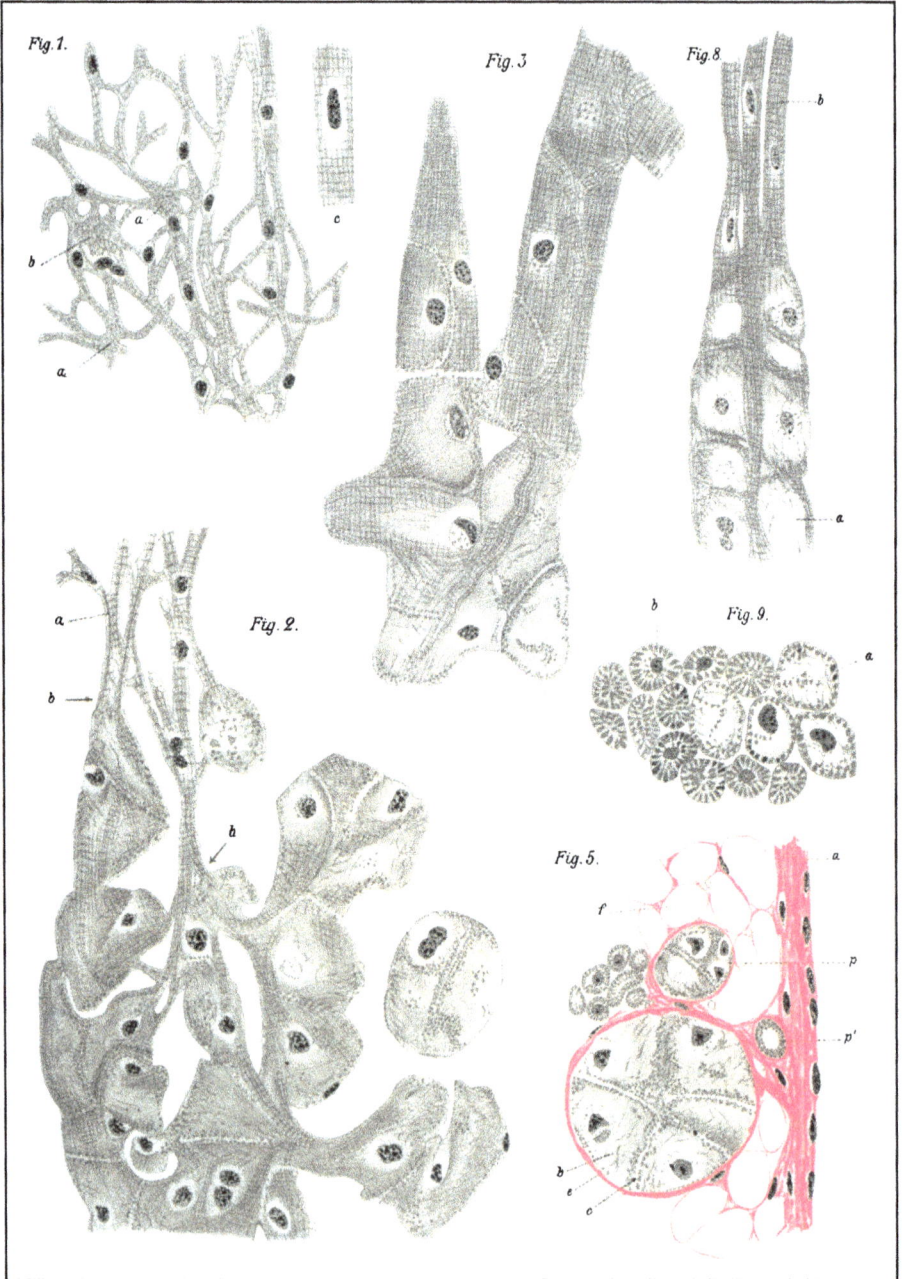

(*continued on next page*)

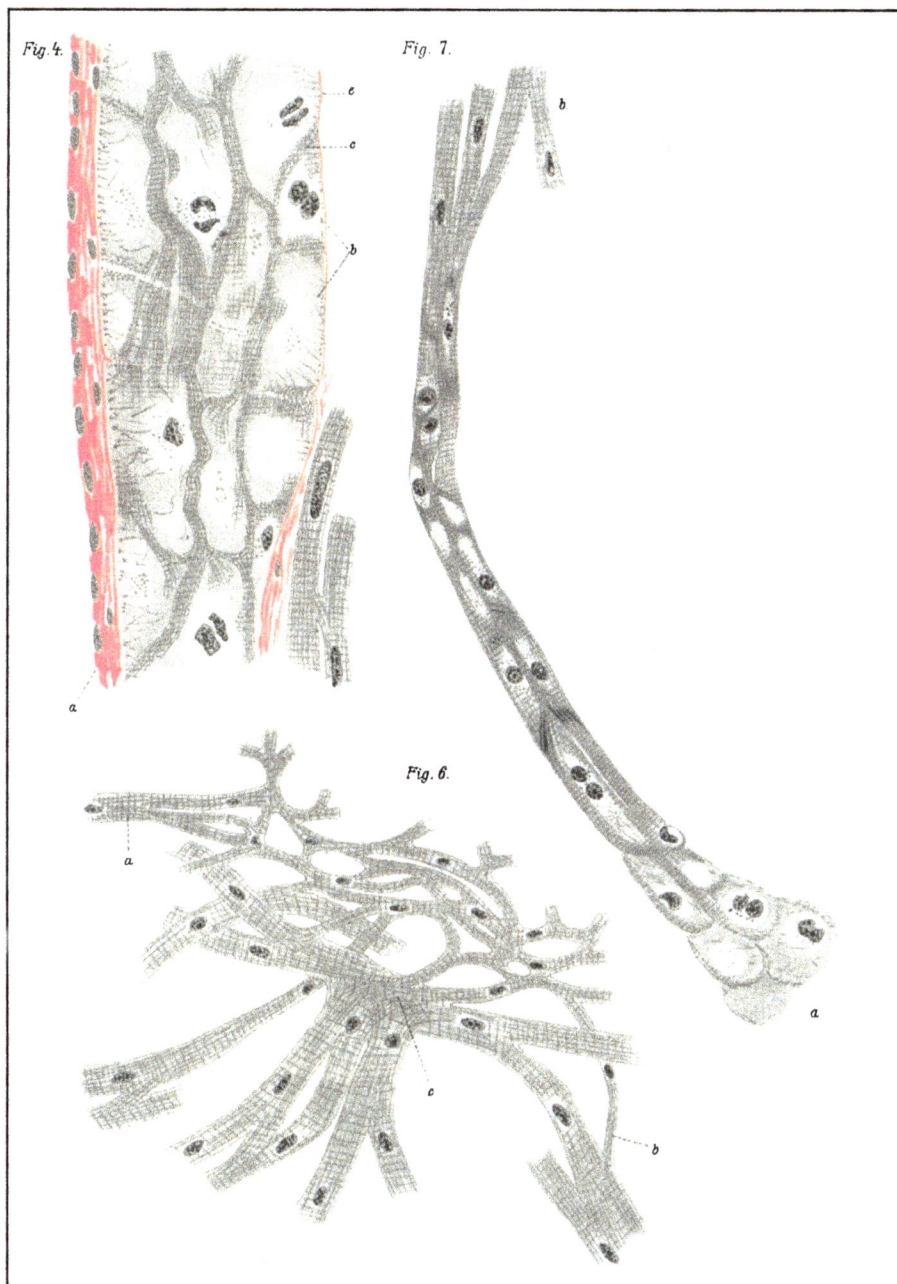

(*continued on next page*)

Histology of the atrioventricular connecting system of the sheep heart

Fig. 1.   Part of the node, i.e. the atrial segment of the connecting system

$a =$ knot point of many muscle fibers

$b =$ cross-sectioned muscle fibers

$c =$ an ordinary atrial muscle fiber (compare the thickness)

Fig. 2.   Part of the transitional portion of the node into the ventricular bundle

$a =$ finer muscle fibers of the node

$b =$ transitions

$c =$ cords of big cells of the ventricular bundle, i.e. cords similar to Purkinje fibers

$d =$ two cross-sectioned big cells lying close side by side

Fig. 3.   Initial portion of the ventricular bundle

Here, more regular cell arrangement is already shown.

Fig. 4.   Longitudinal section of the terminal ramification of the ventricular bundle, i.e. a Purkinje fiber

$a =$ endocardium

$b =$ Purkinje cells

$c =$ cell border

$d =$ ordinary ventricular muscle fibers

$e =$ connective tissue sheath of a Purkinje fiber

Fig. 5.   Cross-sections of three Purkinje fibers of various sizes

$a =$ endocardium

$b =$ Purkinje cells

$c =$ cell borders

$d =$ cross-sections of the ordinary ventricular muscle fibers (compare the thickness)

$e =$ connective tissue sheath of a Purkinje fiber which shows five cells in cross-section

$p =$ a Purkinje fiber consisting of three cells in cross-section

$p' =$ a very small Purkinje fiber which shows only one cell in cross-section

$f =$ subendocardial fatty tissue

Fig. 6.   Transition from the atrial segment of the connecting bundle to the ordinary atrial musculature

$a, b \& c =$ see text (p. 131)

Figs. 7 and 8.   Transition of the terminal fibers of the ventricular bundle to the ordinary ventricular muscle fibers (see text, pp. 131–132); connective tissue sheath is not shown

$a =$ Purkinje fiber

$b =$ ventricular muscle fibers

Fig. 9.   Cross-sections of Purkinje fibers shortly before transition to the ordinary ventricular muscle fibers

surface, sometimes exist in circular arrangements at the periphery of the surface, and sometimes lie divided in several groups. Longitudinally sectioned muscle fibers, therefore, usually demonstrate irregular and nonparallel longitudinal striations, so that the muscle fibers are faintly stained and look threadbare. Most of the cross-striations of the fibers are very faint. The nuclei are oval and shorter than those of the ordinary atrial myocardial cells, while the thickness of the nuclei does not differ. Because the muscle fibers of the network are much thinner than the ordinary atrial muscle fibers, the nuclei look relatively large, so that muscle fibers sometimes swell at the site of a nucleus. The nuclei often lie in a clear halo, and seldom do two nuclei lie close side by side.

These thin muscle fibers run in all possible directions, branching or connecting with others to form a highly irregular and complicated network. The fibers of the network are interwoven one upon the other and side by side. The shape of the meshes of the network is manifold. These meshes are filled with a larger proportion of fatty tissue and a small amount of connective tissue fibers containing numerous small blood vessels and small nerve bundles. Often, two to four thin muscle fibers run for a short distance and then join together into a broad muscle fiber. It is impossible to recognize the border of the fibers, because the fibrils or fibril bundles run from one fiber to the other. The nuclei do not lie on one line in the fused fibers, but are irregularly scattered. This is not the case with the ordinary cardiac muscle fibers. These confluent fibers of the network again separate from each other and participate in the overall formation of the net. Furthermore, it is often observed that four to six, or more, muscle fibers connect with each other in many ways to form a very large star-shaped structure (Fig. 1a). In other words, numerous muscle fibers go out radially from a star-shaped structure and connect with other similar muscle fibers, or with other star-shaped structures. When such a nodal point of numerous muscle fibers is more precisely observed, it is recognized that fibrils with cross-striations, individually or as a bundle, cross over in all directions and run into various muscle fibers radiating from the star. In other words, all of the muscle fibers exchange their fibrils. There are multiple muscle nuclei in such a star-shaped structure, and they are very often surrounded by a clear halo.

The muscle fibers which run more parallel in the initial portion of the atrial segment demonstrate almost the same characteristics as those of the network described above. They are also very thin, and appear to have on average relatively regular and more visible lengthwise and crosswise striations. All of these fibers emerge from the peripheral portion of the network and run in more or less parallel fashion to the posterior. They occasionally connect with each other during their course, but they do not form a distinct network. More connective tissue is seen between each fiber than is the case for the ordinary cardiac musculature.

I divided the atrial segment into two portions, and the only difference worth mentioning is the arrangement of the muscle fibers. The histological characteristics of the individual fibers of both portions are virtually the same. Also, the border between the two portions is not sharply demarcated, and the portion with parallel fibers is sometimes reduced and almost absent. The main mass of the atrial segment is made up of the complicated plexus of small fibers.

This atrial segment of the connecting bundle demonstrates such a characteristic structure not only in its extraordinary thin muscle fibers with very irregular breadths and with very irregular crosswise and lengthwise striations, but also in its highly complicated arrangement of fibers. Because of this, once observed, it can never be mistaken for the ordinary cardiac muscle fibers, because such a peculiar network of muscle fibers appears nowhere else in the sheep heart.

Comment 1. Of course, small muscle fibers also appear elsewhere, for example in the superficial layer of the atrial septum near the attachment line of the septal leaflet of the tricuspid valve. They run more or less parallel in beautiful bundles as seen in the ordinary cardiac muscles, and have no direct relationship with the atrioventricular bundle. I cannot say anything about their significance. A peculiar netlike formation of muscle fibers can also be found in other places, for example, at the junction of the anterior and posterior ventricular walls with the interventricular septum. These nets, however, are composed of the thick ordinary ventricular muscle fibers.

Comment 2. It should also be noted that the illustration (Fig. 1) demonstrating part of the peculiar network is schematic. In reality, the individual small fibers possess more irregular breadths and their cross-striations are usually not so clearly seen as shown in the illustration.

2. *The ventricular segment of the connecting bundle*

This segment begins at the place where the connecting bundle penetrates the atrioventricular fibrocartilaginous septum. It has less histological similarity to the atrial segment and less similarity to the ordinary cardiac musculature. Instead, it shows an interesting and characteristic feature. This segment can also be divided into two portions, i.e. the initial portion and the terminal ramifications; these two portions are histologically different.

(a) The initial portion of the ventricular segment is made up of large and highly peculiar cells. The form of the individual cells is extremely variable. The forms of their sectional surfaces in the fixed preparation are also highly variable. The form is sometimes round, sometimes oval, sometimes triangular, sometimes square, sometimes polygonal and sometimes more narrow and long. The sectional surfaces of the cells often have projections or indentations, and also have multiple irregularities. Likewise, the size of the cells varies a great deal. The cells lie close one after another and, at the same time, two to three, or rarely more, cells lie side by side, forming cell cords. The cords do not usually run straight but as irregular curves. The cords often have side projections, consisting of part of one cell or of an entire cell or of a short process of many cells. Many of the cords run side by side and connect with each other either through the side projections or through direct fusion. They form a highly irregular network (Figs. 2 and 3). This network itself is a considerably large cord surrounded completely by a connective tissue sheath and separated from the adjacent ventricular musculature. The spaces between each cord, i.e. the net meshes, are filled with sparse connective tissue originating from the connective tissue sheath and with relatively rich fatty tissue. In addition, numerous capillaries, small blood vessels and small nerve bundles run through the spaces. Individual cell cords are also surrounded with a very fine connective tissue sheath.

When a cord is observed at stronger magnification in its longitudinal section, the cells constituting the cord are seen to show length and cross-striations. These striations often spread equally all over the cell surfaces. In most cases, nonetheless, they appear distinctly only at the border of cells lying side by side. In the latter situation, the fibril groups belonging to both cells and usually running in a strong wave appear at first to be one bundle. When such fibril bundles are precisely examined, a dark or clear line, and not seldom a narrow fine gap, is often recognized running lengthwise in the middle of the bundle. This line or gap indicates the border between the two neighboring cells. This situation can be much better observed at the cross-sectioned cell cords. The sectional surfaces of the fibrils usually appear like fine points which can be seen most distinctly at the margins of the neighboring cells. The points are sometimes sparsely scattered in the entire sectional surface, and sometimes densely gathered at a certain point. From these findings, it is concluded that the large cells have cross-striated fibrils which are best distinguished at the periphery, i.e. the border of the neighboring cells, and that the fibrils sometimes appear at the inner portion of the cells. Usually the fibrils run along the same direction of the long axis of the cord. It is concluded, therefore, that each cell is also arranged in parallel fashion to the direction of the cord. As the cell cords run irregularly, and have bendings or even processes, cross-sectioned cells are not infrequently observed close beside longitudinally sectioned cells. Fibril bundles continue from one cell to another without interruption, as can be observed especially well in longitudinally sectioned cords.

These cell cords were stained so densely and so opaque that, in some of them, I was not able to recognize any finer structure. (All of these preparations were nine microns thick.) I further noticed that, sometimes, only a certain part of the cell, either its center, its periphery or its border area, was stained with varying intensity. When a site intensively stained was precisely examined, it was usually found that here the fibrils were especially well developed. Now, it is uncertain whether this dense staining of the cells is due to a particular characteristic of the cells or is just an artifact. Both assumptions are possible, because this portion was located in the middle of the thick ventricular septum and, therefore, fixation might have been ineffective in the central part of the septum which was not fixed long enough in Formol-Müller, when compared with the subendocardial area. Had I examined this portion in its fresh condition, I would have obtained much more reliable findings. Unfortunately, I must refrain from this attempt because the study is very difficult, if not absolutely impossible, due to the inner position of the portion. Nevertheless, it seems to me certain that individual cells of this portion possess, on average, more fibrils than the cells of the subsequent portion, i.e. the terminal ramifications. Concerning nuclei, there is no difference between in the cells of this portion and in the terminal ramifications. Later, I will describe them together.

Now, I would like to make a comment about the transition from the atrial to the ventricular segment. This transition occurs suddenly just at the border between the atrial and the ventricular septum in a highly characteristic way. The large cells at the initial portion of the ventricular segment give forth one, rarely two or three thin muscle fibers from their free surfaces facing the atrium or rarely from their side surfaces. These thin muscle fibers are nothing but the above-mentioned muscle fibers of the atrial segment forming a net in a complicated way. When the transition of the thin fibers of the atrial bundle to the thick fibers of the ventricular bundle is precisely observed, it is recognized that the bundles of fibrils of the small fibers continuously run into the large muscle fibers. I sketched part of the transition (Fig. 2). You can see from this sketch how abruptly this transition occurs.

As I have already mentioned in the chapter on anatomy, the thick fibers making up the network of the initial portion of the ventricular segment remind me, at first glance, of the well-known Purkinje fibers of the ventricular inner surface. The fact that all of the authors investigating the so-called Purkinje fibers in the sheep heart have failed until now to see the fibers at this site is easily explained. Because the network is found at the middle uppermost part of the ventricular septum, little attention might have been aroused in the former investigators. The fibers are not completely similar to Purkinje fibers, but they gradually change to become them. These differentiated special fibers composing a network at the initial portion of the ventricular segment can be traced further downward until they bifurcate into the left and right bundle branches, and to the initial portions of both these bundle branches.

Now follows the second portion of the ventricular segment to the initial portion. It comprises most of both the bundle branches and all of the terminal ramifications known for a long time as the so-called Purkinje fibers.

The transition from the initial ventricular portion to the second portion takes place so gradually that it is difficult to make a definite border. If both of the bundle branches are traced downward, the opaque and large cells gradually become transparent. In the left bundle branch, this occurs approximately at the place where the bundle reaches the subendocardium. In the sheep heart, the right bundle branch usually does not reach the endocardium. The bundle branch, however, gradually approaches the endocardium and finally enters the trabecular cord described in detail in the anatomical chapter. During its course, the cells change their properties and take on the typical characteristics of Purkinje cells.

(b) As I have already described in detail in the anatomical chapter, I will not repeat how both of the bundle branches and their terminal ramifications take their courses and spread all over the inner surfaces of the right and left ventricles. I will describe only the histology of the terminal ramifications of the system.

As described above, the cell cords of the initial ventricular portion have rough projections and indentations. The gaps between cell cords, i.e. the net meshes, are relatively wide and highly irregular. As the cells become more transparent, the thickness of the cell cords gradually becomes more even; the cords become more round and run more parallel than before. Accordingly, the gaps between cell cords become thinner and longer, whereby the diameter of both the bundle branches becomes smaller. When Purkinje cells show all their characteristics, the cell cords usually have a regular and round form. Many more cell cords run side by side in both the bundle branches and, during their courses, the cords often divide or connect with each other, forming a long stretched net inside a common connective tissue sheath. The net is somewhat looser in the left bundle branch than in the right. Also in this portion, the meshes are usually filled with fatty tissue, connective tissue fibers, small blood vessels, capillaries and several small nerve bundles. Each cell cord has its own thin connective tissue sheath. Both the bundle branches become the terminal ramifications in this fashion.

In the chapter on topographical anatomy, I have already described precisely how the cell cords, during their courses either in tendinous fiber-like connective tissue cords or in the subendocardium, branch and spread or connect with other cords in a very interesting way so as to form nets everywhere. Further, I have already mentioned that the terminal ramifications not only exist in the subendocardium but also enter the myocardium accompanied by subendocardial connective tissue fibers. I also described the macroscopic appearance of the subendocardial terminal ramifications and the extent to which they can be traced. I will not repeat these descriptions here.

Individual cell cords of the terminal ramifications are mostly round. They are often, however, irregularly formed and, on occasion, take the form of a broad plate or band. The cords are composed of cells lying close side by side, or one after another. There are usually 3–6 cells in cross section. Rarely, the number of the cells is smaller, occasionally more, up to 40–50 cells being seen side by side. The size of the cords varies markedly, according to the number of cells lying side by side. However, it is not always proportional to the number of cells. When there are numerous cells the size is relatively small, because, on the average, individual cells are smaller than usual in such cases.

In fixed preparations, the form of each cell in cross section is markedly variable. It may be round, oval, semilunar, triangular, quadrangular or polygonal. Similarly, the cells show all possible forms when sectioned lengthwise. They usually extend in the direction of the cord. Occasionally, they are wider than long. Individual cells are very large, but their sizes vary a great deal. Those different forms can be well recognized in curetting fresh preparations.

The finer structure, not only of the cord but also of each cell, has been described before in various fashions by many authors who made detailed investigations of Purkinje fibers. The main controversy has been whether the fiber is composed of only one kind of cells or of two morphologically different cells. The latter viewpoint was energetically supported by v. Heßling, Lehnert and Schmalz. Most other authors opposed this viewpoint. (Compare the literature on Purkinje fibers cited later!) How can the different viewpoints be reconciled?

When the cords are seen at weak magnification, they are divided into many fields of various forms and sizes by relatively broad and dim, darkly stained lines. Each field is a territory of a cell or, in other words, a corn[*], as named by many authors. These dark lines, however, are not seen in all cells, nor at all sides of a cell. The lines are almost always absent at the externally facing free side of those cells which lie at the rim of a cord and are absent here and there even inside the cell cords. When such a cord is observed at stronger magnification, groups of cross-striated fibrils with a relatively regular breadth and a sharp boundary are observed at the sites of

---

[*]*Zell-bezw. Kornterritorium*

the dark lines. The groups of fibrils usually form a net through branching and unifying, and thus divide the cord into many polygonal fields. These fields — in other words, the meshes of the net — appear somewhat hyalinous and have one to two, or seldom three, nuclei in each field. In addition, pigment granules, fatty droplets and other granulous deposits are seen in this hyalinous mass. Because these groups of cross-striated fibrils which form the net are markedly different in most instances to the hyalinous mass, i.e. cells or corns, v. Heßling, Schmalz and others made the assumption that there were two different components. v. Heßling differentiated corns from the nets of cross-striated fibril groups ("intersubstance"). On the other hand, Schmalz recognized two components, i.e. peculiar netlike fibrillar muscle substance and special cells lying in the nets.

First of all, the question is raised whether the fibril groups run outside or inside the cells. When an endocardial fragment of the fresh ventricle of the fresh sheep heart is detached from the site where Purkinje fibers are macroscopically seen, and the fragment facing the myocardium is scratched with a knife or a needle, not only Purkinje fibers but also frequently their cells are obtained. The size and form of the individual cells are markedly different, as mentioned before. When these isolated or still connected cells are observed precisely by sliding up and down the cylinder of a microscope at strong magnification, the cross-striated fibrils are observed to be running regularly on the surface of the hyalinous cells. Even by a minimal change in the height of the cylinder, the fibrils can be made to disappear very easily. The fibrils run from one end of the cell to the other, and the cross-striations run vertically to the direction of the fibrils. Occasionally, there are isolated cells in which fibrils exist not all over the surface, but only at a side margin of the cells. More or less similar findings are obtained in a longitudinally sectioned cell cord of a fixed preparation. In those preparations, as with fresh examinations, it can be confirmed that fibrils usually run parallel to, and correspondingly the cross-striations run vertical to, the long axis of the cell cord, as is usually the case. Sometimes, the cells lie in somewhat different directions, although not so strongly deviated as in the initial portion of the ventricular segment. Usually, the fibrils of all the cells are not observed at the same time in one microscopical field, because the cells lie at various heights. When the fibril groups mentioned above, seemingly running between individual cells and containing the cells inside their meshes, are precisely observed, it is recognized that they are especially well-seen cross-striated fibrils and extend a long distance in a longitudinal direction without noticeable interruption of the fibrils. The fibril groups seem to be sharply demarcated on their sides. However, they are the above-mentioned bundles or groups of fibrils which are seen on the cell surfaces. This is confirmed by moving the microscopic cylinder upward and downward. Moreover, individual fibrils or small bundles of fibrils enter not infrequently the interior of a cell and extend in various directions through the cell or spread in a fan shape, so that a sharp border between the homogeneous cell body and the fibrils cannot always be confirmed in a longitudinally sectioned cell cord (Fig. 4). The cell borders, therefore, do not lie between the fibrils and the hyalinous mass, but these two elements belong together to the same component. The cell border must be sought at another site. As a matter of fact, by manipulating the height of the cylinder, a distinct and sharp line, sometimes shiny and sometimes dark, can usually be recognized in the midst of the groups of individual fibrils in their longitudinal directions. Obermeier noticed and described this line, but Lehnert argued wrongly against him. This line must be regarded as a cell border, and the group of fibrils must be divided into two parts belonging to the adjacent cells. I was unable to reproduce naturally all these border lines in Fig. 4.

How do these groups of fibrils appear in the cross-sectioned cell cords? This situation can be seen much better in cross-section (Fig. 5). At this section of the cell cords, the cut ends of individual fibrils are fine granules of various sizes and forms. Larger granules seem to represent the cross-section not of only one fibril, but of many fibrils. These granules are generally seen in one or two relatively regular layers at the outermost periphery of individual cells, and usually only at the sites of the cells facing the adjacent cells. For example, when a cell lies in the middle of a large cell cord, and is bordered by other cells from all sides, the cell has granules, i.e. cross-sectioned fibrils, throughout its periphery. When a cell is situated at the periphery of a cell cord, granules are usually absent at the side of the cell wall making up the outer surface of the cord. This arrangement of fibrils is the rule, although there are deviations. There are often fibrils also at the side of the cell wall just mentioned. In addition, fibrils exist in a small group or are sparsely scattered inside a cell body.

The layer of the fibril at the border of a cell facing others sometimes changes its thickness and arrangement. The outermost fibril layer of individual cells is usually arranged regularly, though at times in a wavy line. The other layers of fibrils close behind the outermost layer, if any, are mostly in a more irregular form. It is, therefore, impossible to draw a sharp border between the fibril layer and the hyalinous cell body. When the border of two adjacent cells is observed precisely, a narrow clear line is almost always seen between the outermost lines of granules of the two cells. This is nothing but the border between the two cells. All the fibrils must exist inside the cells. Otherwise, a border must be seen in cross-section between the layer of fibrils and the hyalinous cell body. The viewpoint of v. Heßling and Schmalz, that Purkinje fibers consist of homogeneous cells and muscle fibers, can therefore no longer be justified. On the contrary, it seems to me certain that Purkinje fibers are composed exclusively of one morphological entity, i.e. large cells usually possessing differentiated fibrils at their periphery.

The cell body of individual larger cells is composed of a transparent, hyalinous and undifferentiated protoplasmic mass and of cross-striated fibrils usually running only at the periphery of the cells, and seldom inside the protoplasm. Fibrils run parallel to the longitudinal direction of the cell cords. In addition to these major fibrils, numerous more-or-less fine fibrils, or small bundles of fibrils, are further recognized in most of the cells. They branch from the longitudinal bundles of fibrils and run irregularly in various directions in the homogeneous protoplasm. In rare cases, these irregular fibrils exist in a great number, and strongly mask the homogeneous appearance of the cell body, as the fibrils lie in layers one upon the other or in confused clusters. All these fibrils have the characteristics of the fibrils of the ordinary cardiac muscle fibers, as can be shown by using various reagents.

The cells have one to two, and sometimes three, nuclei surrounded by a clear halo of various forms. In fixed and stained preparations, a nuclear halo is usually sharply demarcated by protoplasmic masses, and almost always contains fatty droplet gaps, yellow pigments and not infrequently numerous dark lumpy substances of various sizes and forms. The significance of the substances is unknown to me. The nuclei are large, and often their forms are round, oval, polygonal, semilunar or kidney-shaped. When there are two or three nuclei in one cell, they usually lie close together one after another, mostly in the direction of the long axis of the cell cord. There are also cases where two nuclei lie distantly in one cell. When there are two kidney-shaped nuclei, they usually face each other across their concave sides. Numerous small bodies are clearly recognized in the nuclei.

When the cells form a cord by lying close side by side and one after another, individual fibrils run not only in one cell territory, but also continuously from one cell to the other. The borders between the cell territories lying one after the other consequently become concealed and inconspicuous, as do the longitudinal borders between individual fibril groups, which I explained before. Here, a question is raised whether there is no longitudinal continuity of the cells in Purkinje fibers, as with the ordinary cardiac muscle fibers. In fact, there is no continuity of the cells in Purkinje fibers. By using the Mallory method or a silver solution, fine borders between territories of the cells lying one after the other or side by side are easily demonstrated. Moreover, apparent splits between the cells, constantly bridged by fibrils, are sometimes recognized. There is continuity of fibrils but no continuity of protoplasm. There is a similar situation; Schridde[11] recently illustrated more clearly the continuity of fibrils in cells of the epidermis.

As bundles of fibrils running on cell borders connect with each other, directly proceed from one cell territory to the other, and further penetrate through individual cells, the fibrils form an extremely complicated net spreading over many cells without any interruptions.

In another feature, Purkinje fibers essentially differ from the ordinary cardiac musculature. As individual fibers of the ordinary cardiac musculature are surrounded everywhere in their longitudinal direction by the finest connective tissue fibers, the individual fibers are isolated up to the site of bridgelike connections. On the other hand, in Purkinje fibers, each of the cell bundles is surrounded by a common connective tissue sheath, as illustrated in Figs. 4 and 5. The connective tissue sheath here and there sends septums into the bundle, making indentations and constrictions on its surface. The bundle is, however, nowhere separated into individual cells. Individual Purkinje cells are intimately connected with each other. The absence of a separating net of connective tissue and of capillaries facilitates the multiple connections and crossings of the system of fibrils.

For the reason mentioned above, a Purkinje fiber, whether thick or thin, corresponds to one muscle fiber, i.e. a primitive bundle of the ordinary cardiac musculature.

I cannot explain why fibrils develop best at the periphery of a cell body, especially at the site of a cell border. This is a peculiar characteristic not only of these cells but also of all the muscle fibers of the connecting system. This will be shown later in the description of the developmental stages of the system in dogs and humans.

Now, I describe the remarkable segments of the connecting system, namely the transitional zones. In the sheep, there are three important transitions, of which only one was formerly recognized by the investigators of the Purkinje fibers. The three transitions are (1) the transition between the ordinary atrial musculature and the atrial segment of the connecting system; (2) the transition between the terminal ramifications of the ventricular segment and the ordinary ventricular musculature; and (3) the transition between the atrial segment and the ventricular segment. Of these three transitions, I have already explained in detail the transition between the atrial and the ventricular segment. Here, therefore, I will describe precisely the first and the second transition.

The connections between the atrial segment and the ordinary atrial musculature take place mainly at the posterior periphery of the atrial segment. It is noteworthy, however, that not all of the fibers of the atrial segment connect with the ordinary atrial muscle fibers. In contrast, many fibers of the atrial segment end without connection in the abundant fatty tissue usually found in this region. I cannot insist on this with absolute certainty, because the preparations of the two sheep hearts were not of continuous series, but rather of staged sections, as mentioned earlier. Be that as it may, the posterior end of the connecting system was bordered mostly by thick fatty tissue on its left, posterior, superior and inferior aspects. This fatty tissue lies in the middle of the atrial septum, and the muscle fibers run through the fatty tissue to scatter in various directions. Therefore, the posterior extent of the node is bordered only at its right side by the atrial musculature. Accordingly, the connection between the fibers of the connecting system and the ordinary atrial musculature is usually seen only at this site.

The mode of connection varies. Either two or three thin fibers running relatively parallel or branching directly from the complicated net join together to form a broader atrial muscle fiber (Fig. 6, *a*), or a thin fiber connects directly with the side surface of a neighboring ordinary atrial fiber (Fig. 6, *b*). The fibrils continuously run into the ordinary atrial fibers, as is always the case with the ordinary myocardium when its fibers connect together. Furthermore — and this seems to be characteristic — a peculiar arrangement of individual atrial fibers can often be seen. These are the atrial muscle fibers which do not run parallel in a bundle but come separately from various directions, as described earlier in the case of heart No. 155, and join together often to make a considerable star form (Fig. 6, *c*). Thin muscle fibers of the connecting bundle are more likely to join to this star form. When the thin muscle fibers are observed precisely, it is recognized that the fibrils in the star form run in various directions by crossing each other. It is presumed that individual fibrils of the connecting bundle run into many atrial fibers of the star form, and that the fibrils further spread in various directions through the atrial fibers which run more or less radially. All these transitions are drawn as naturally as possible in Fig. 6. The contour of the individual fibers of the connecting bundle is, however, illustrated too schematically.

The transition from the terminal ramification of the connecting bundle to the ordinary ventricular muscle fibers: these transitions are found everywhere scattered over the whole ventricular musculature, and especially frequently in the subendocardial regions. In the myocardium, they usually happen only at the inner two-thirds of the parietal wall, and at the left and right superficial layers of the septum. The transition occurs infrequently in the middle of the septum and at the outer one-third of the parietal wall. I have never seen transitions of Purkinje fibers in the subepicardium of my preparations. This finding is in contrast with the statements of v. Heßling and Hofmann. As far as the regional frequency of transitions in the heart is concerned, I believe that the transitions occur most frequently at both the papillary muscles and the apical portion of the left ventricle, and only scarcely at the upper portion of the septum. All the transitions are localized in accordance with the situation of the course and branching of the terminal ramifications of the system.

The transitions occur not at the main cords, but at their terminal ramifications, either in the subendocardium or only after the ramifications have entered the myocardium.

The transition of the terminal ramifications of the connecting system to the ordinary cross-striated cardiac muscle fibers takes place in various ways. Generally, it takes place as follows. Firstly, individual cells of the terminal ramifications, which are as a rule thin, and in which only two cells are usually recognized lying side by side when seen in a longitudinal section, become longer and thinner. Both pole rims, as well as side rims of the cells, more or less irregularly round previously, become gradually straighter. At the same time, the transparency of the cells is reduced. This change is more apparent in the cells lying more distally. Individual cells become thinner and are stretched lengthwise. The central hyalinous mass is gradually reduced and peripheral longitudinal and cross-striations become more distinct and regular. Simultaneously, therefore, transparency of the cells is gradually reduced. Further, the cells, no longer different from the ordinary cardiac muscle fibers, continue and connect with the ordinary cardiac muscles. This is a typical mode of connection. This transition occurs so gradually that it is difficult to recognize any certain border between the cell cords and the cardiac muscle fibers. The length of the transitional zone, if it is thus called, varies markedly. In some situations it is long, and in others it is very short. In the former situation, after the long stretched cells, short cells sometimes succeed. Two illustrations show how this transition occurs in a longitudinal section (Figs. 7 and 8). Further, a cross-sectional illustration just before the transition is shown (Fig. 9). Here, the cells are already much smaller, their central hyalinous substances are reduced and the peripheral fibrils are increased.

Hofmann insisted that, as shown by one of his illustrations (Fig. 1 of his study), Purkinje fibers connect not only in one direction but sometimes in both directions with the cardiac muscle fibers. This means that Purkinje fibers may appear to be inserted in the course of the cardiac muscle fibers. I do not doubt that Hofmann saw such a microscopical finding, although I could not confirm this phenomenon in my numerous preparations. Here, I will emphasize this point, because from my viewpoint this phenomenon is not of meaningless physiological significance of Purkinje fibers. Terminal ramifications of Purkinje fibers branch in many twigs and connect with the cardiac muscle fibers. The directions are quite varied. Branching from the stem of the ramification, the twigs take courses at acute, right and obtuse angles, and even take reversed courses. The directions are usually very irregular and only seldom straight for a short extent. When a situation occurs such that a terminal twig finally branches opposite to two twigs in a straight line on one plane and, further that incidentally a cut surface is exactly on this line and on the same plane, the illustration shown by Hofmann will be obtained. A preparation of only one section is not enough to prove that a piece of Purkinje fiber is inserted without any connection with other Purkinje fibers between cardiac muscle fibers. This situation can only be determined by continuous serial sections. I do not know whether Hofmann precisely examined this possibility by serial sections. Anyway, I understand the illustration not in his sense but from my viewpoint that two terminal twigs run exactly in opposite directions to each other. When Hofmann's illustration is precisely examined, a narrow portion is seen almost in the middle of the Purkinje fiber. This portion can, from my viewpoint, be taken as a branching portion from a stem to two twigs.

In the sheep heart, although seldom seen, there is another mode of transition. The transition occurs not in thin fibers as stated above, but in broad bundles. In sheep heart No. 160, I have seen this mode of transition especially well in the subendocardium at the superoposterior portion of the ventricular septum, near the attachment of the aortic leaflet of the mitral valve. A great number of Purkinje fibers, lying irregularly one upon the other, side by side and one after the other, gradually take on a more regular arrangement. The cell borders become straighter and the cell bodies longer and thinner. The fibrils are more distinctly seen and, accordingly, the hyalinous mass is reduced. The nuclei gradually become longer. In this way, this large group of Purkinje cells, as a whole, connects with a group of the ordinary cardiac muscle fibers, or Purkinje cells lying previously close side by side form a group of many short cell cords lying close side by side, and soon connect with the ordinary cardiac muscle fibers in the mode described above. This transition, in which a large group of cells connects, as a closed mass, with the ordinary cardiac muscle fibers through a short transitional zone, appears unique. In principle, however, it is the same as the thin fiber transitions mentioned before.

I would like to make a further comment on *the connective tissue sheath of the connecting system.* The initial portion of the ventricular bundle, and both its bundle branches, have two kinds of connective tissue sheath: a common sheath and a sheath for individual cords. The common sheath surrounds the entire connecting bundle, including its branches, and separates it from the adjacent ventricular musculature. The common sheath consists of relatively loose connective tissue fibers and elastic tissue. The sheath is relatively thick and has no layers. The connective tissue fibers join with the adjacent interstitial connective tissue fibers of the myocardium or of blood vessels. When the connecting bundle reaches the subendo-cardium, the common sheath consists of subendocardial connective tissue fibers and shows large gaps, so that it is no longer possible to call it a closed sheath. The connective tissue sheaths surrounding individual cell cords are usually thin, and follow every unevenness of the surface of the cords. However, they do not penetrate inside the cell cord. Individual cells, therefore, come into contact with the sheath only at their free surfaces. In the common sheath, many small blood vessels, and capillaries, as well as small nerve bundles are seen, which enter the sheaths of the individual cell cords.

The terminal ramifications of the connecting bundle, i.e. individual Purkinje fibers, also have a more or less thick connective tissue sheath. When Purkinje fibers lie in the subendocardium, the sheath is made up of loose subendocardial connective tissue. When the terminal ramifications enter the myocardium, the subendocardial connective tissue accompanies them as sheath material. The sheaths are multiply laminar. The inner surface of the sheath follows exactly the surface of the corresponding cell cord, and the sheath often sends short septums into the cell cord. These circumstances are well recognized in fixed preparations. As the result of shrinkage of the cell cord, a narrow, or seldom a wide gap is often made between the cell cord and the sheath — a phenomenon especially well recognized in the suben-docardial cell cords. When these sites are precisely observed, it is seen that processes or indentations of the inner surface of the sheath exactly fit the outer surface of the corresponding cell cord. This phenomenon in fixed preparations, as well as the fact that individual cells and even cell cords fall down nakedly by scratching in fresh preparations, indicates that connec-tions between the cord and its sheath are relatively loose.

The connective tissue sheath has many nuclei and blood capillaries. The connective tissue fibers themselves connect with interstitial connective tissue fibers of the adjacent cardiac musculature.

At the transitional zone from Purkinje fibers to the ordinary cardiac muscle fibers, the sheaths of Purkinje fibers gradually become thinner and finally connect with the perimysium of the cardiac muscle fibers.

(b) *Dog heart*

The system in the dog is not as sharply separated histologically from the ordinary cardiac musculature as in the sheep. Nevertheless, the muscle fibers of the system can be relatively well differentiated not only topographically and anatomically but also histologically from the ordinary cardiac muscle fibers. The system is also divided histologically into the atrial and the ventricular segment. The transition between the two segments, however, is gradual, and this gradual transition is a difference between the systems of dog and sheep.

1. *The atrial segment of the connecting system*

This segment can also be divided, with regard to fiber arrangement, into two portions as in the sheep, namely the anterior net-forming portion and the posterior, more parallelly arranged portion. The two portions together constitute a long spindle form as already described, and are almost completely surrounded by fatty tissue on the superior, left and inferior sides. The amount of fatty tissue, however, varies markedly in individual hearts. In a newborn dog, fatty tissue is almost entirely absent.

(a) The anterior spindle-shaped portion of the atrial segment is characterized by the fact that it consists of a dense network of muscle fibers. Here, the muscle fibers are stained much paler than the rest of the atrium. Although there are longitudinal and cross-striations, the cross-striation is so unclear and faint that it is sometimes difficult to be recognized in several muscle fibers. In all fibers, longitudinal striations are usually well recognized, although sparse in number. In cross-sectional surfaces of the individual muscle fibers, a smaller number of fibrils and a

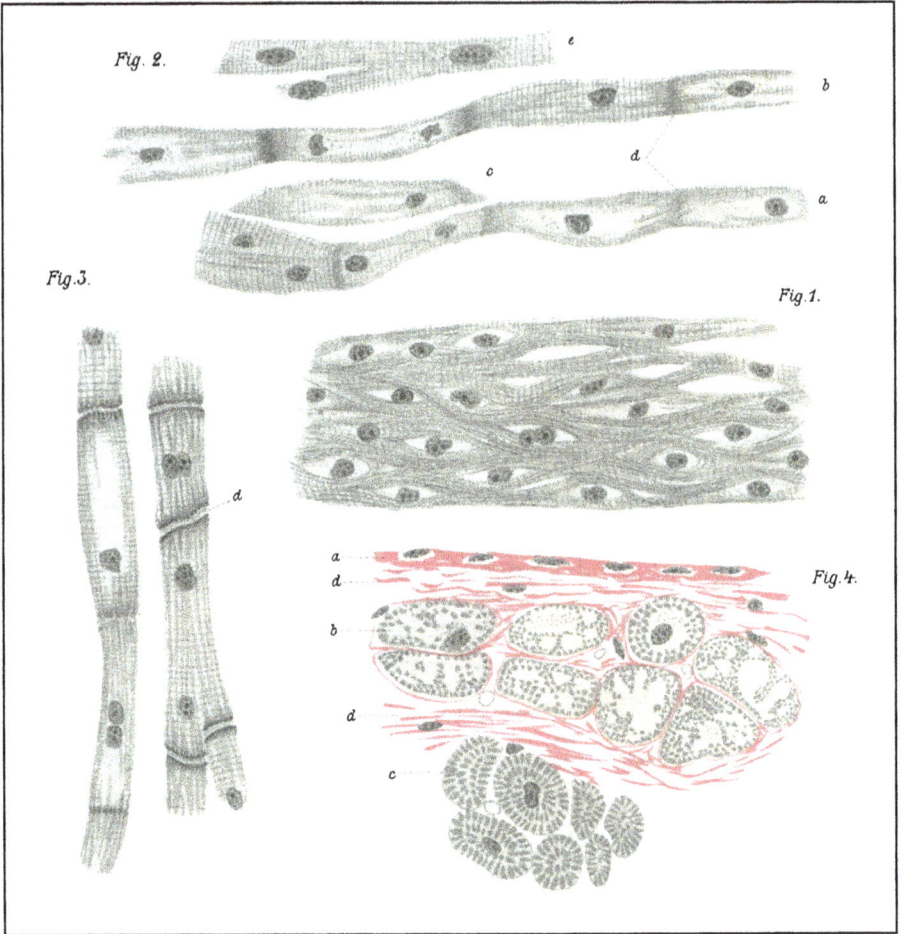

Histology of the atrioventricular connecting system of the dog heart

Fig. 1. Characteristic muscle complex in the upper course of the ventricular bundle

Figs. 2 & 3. Muscle fibers of the terminal ramifications of the ventricular bundle, i.e. Purkinje fibers of the dog heart

  a, b & *c* = individual muscle fibers of the terminal ramifications

    d = cross-bands (cell border?)

    e = ordinary ventricular muscle fiber

(continued on next page)

(continued from previous page)

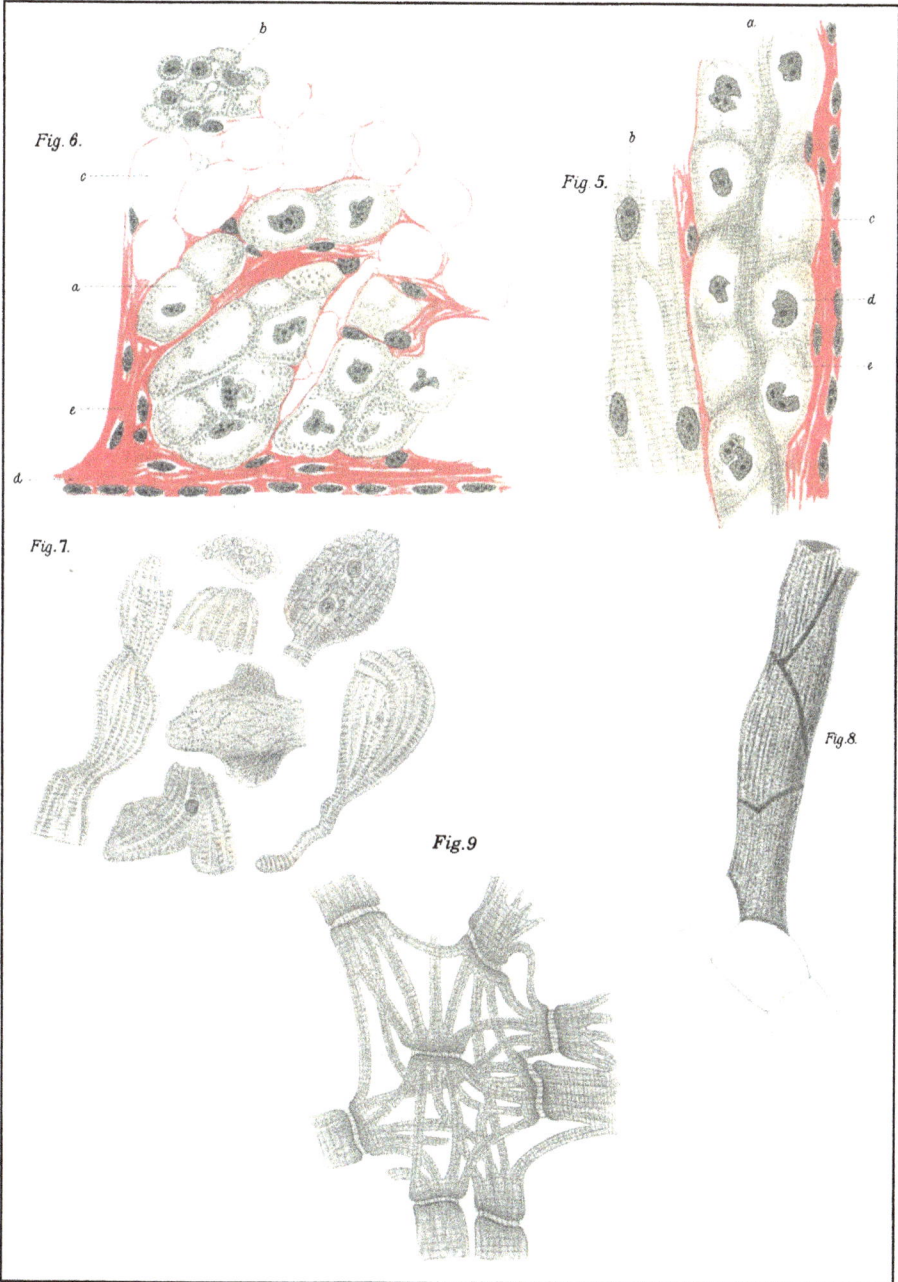

Fig. 6.

Fig. 5.

Fig. 7.

Fig. 8.

Fig. 9

Fig. 4. Cross-section of the terminal ramifications of the ventricular bundle
  a = endocardium
  b = cross-sectioned Purkinje fibers
  c = cross-sectioned ordinary ventricular muscle fibers
  d = subendocardial connective tissue

Fig. 5. A longitudinally sectioned Purkinje fiber of a three-day-old dog
  a = a Purkinje fiber which shows still well a cell border
  b = ordinary ventricular muscle fibers, in which longitudinal striations are seen to be
      sparse and delicate, while cross-striations are highly visible
  c, *d*, *e*, etc. = individual Purkinje cells

Fig. 6. Cross-sectioned Purkinje fibers of the same dog
  a = Purkinje cells
  b = cross-sectioned ordinary ventricular muscle fibers having sparse fibrils
  c = fatty tissue
  d = endocardium
  e = subendocardial connective tissue fibers accompanying Purkinje fibers

Fig. 7. Reproduction of Schmaltz's illustration; see text, pp. 149–150

Fig. 8. Reproduction of Obermeier's illustration; see text, p. 150

**Fig. 9. Characteristic exchange of fibril bundles among individual muscle fibers of
    various Purkinje fibers (compare with text, p. 148)**

greater amount of protoplasm are distinctly recognized when compared with the ordinary atrial muscle fibers. The fibrils are arranged irregularly. They lie neither exclusively at the periphery of the muscle fibers as seen in an embryonal heart, nor distributed evenly in the fibers as is the case in the ordinary cardiac muscle fibers. Rather, they lie scattered irregularly in the protoplasm. Accordingly, in longitudinally sectioned muscle fibers, irregular gaps are observed between each group of fibrils. This sparsity of fibrils is the reason why the fibers are stained palely. The nuclei are variously sized, differently shaped and have clear small bodies. Some of the nuclei are beautifully oval or round, some spindle-shaped, and some very long and thin. Most of them, however, have a manifold and polygonal shape, not seldom representing "Leistenkerne."* Generally, the nuclei are characterized as thicker and shorter than those of the ordinary atrial muscle fibers, where longish oval nuclei are predominantly seen. But all possible differently

---

*Nuclei showing ridges on their surfaces.

shaped nuclei can be seen sporadically. Usually there is only one nucleus, seldom two, and rarely three lying close side by side.

The thickness varies in individual muscle fibers. Moreover, even one fiber often shows thick and thin portions during its short course. On the average, the fibers are thinner than the ordinary atrial muscle fibers, although not so thin as those of the sheep.

Branching or connecting with others, the peculiar muscle fibers run in various directions and form an interrelated and complicated network. Individual fibrils, or bundles of fibrils, continuously run from one muscle fiber to the other. The connecting sites, i.e. the knot points of radiating muscle fibers, are usually much broader than the individual muscle fibers. Not seldom, four or five muscle fibers meet in a knot point. The knot takes on a star shape, where the fibrils, crossing each other in a very complicated way, run from one muscle fiber to the other. Net meshes are usually narrow and take on many shapes. They are often round or oval. Accordingly, the individual muscle fibers connect with each other at obtuse angles. The network as a whole looks somewhat different from that of the sheep heart described earlier. In the sheep heart, except for a number of large star-shaped knots, threads of the net mostly consist of small individual muscle fibers, and the meshes of the net are relatively wide. In the dog, the meshes are usually narrow. The knot points and the individual muscle fibers lie so close side by side that the meshes are difficult to see in several sites. In the adult dog, the tightness of the muscle networks often appears so clearly that this portion of the connecting bundle can easily be differentiated from the ordinary cardiac musculature even at weak magnification. The portion is further characterized by its relatively abundant connective tissue originating from the atrioventricular fibrous septum. Due to the abundant connective tissue, this portion is stained strongly reddish in a van Gieson preparation. For simplicity, I will call this portion of the atrial segment, i.e. the network, the "node."

Muscle fibers continue from this node both forward and backward, so that it is difficult to confirm a definite boundary for the node.

(b) The backward continuation forms the posterior portion of the atrial segment of the connecting bundle. These muscle fibers originate not only from the posterior end of the node, but also from the sides, especially the right side, of the posterior half of the node. Here, the individual muscle fibers are very thin. They do not make a complicated network but run more parallel and posteriorly, usually not isolated but arranged in many small bundles. The fibers are separated from each other here by abundant connective tissue. The bundles usually consist of closely pressed muscle fibers, so that a border between the muscle fibers is difficult to confirm with precision. The fibers also have not only longitudinal but also cross-striations. The striations, however, are not seen so clearly and beautifully as are those in the ordinary cardiac muscle fibers. Here, the fibrils are sparse, as in the fibers of the node, and are arranged irregularly. The preponderance of protoplasm over fibrils, which was seen very clearly in the node, is reduced in these muscle fibers. Nuclei are usually oval or of longish spindle shape, but also show irregular shapes. There are more nuclei here than in the ordinary atrial muscle fibers. In contrast, double nuclei, often seen in the fibers of the node, are hardly observed here. As the nuclei are not so small, and as the muscle fibers are usually thin, the nuclei often occupy the whole width of the muscle fibers, or else the muscle fibers are swollen at the sites of the nuclei. As stated before, the thin muscle fibers are arranged in many small and firm bundles and run posteriorly in almost horizontal and parallel fashion approximately up to the floor of the coronary sinus. Connective tissue is abundant between individual bundles. Penetrating in between individual muscle fibers, connective tissue surrounds the fibers like perimysium. This portion of the atrial segment, consisting of muscle fibers running in parallel fashion, connects with the ordinary atrial muscle fibers. As the connecting bundle is situated close to the atrial musculature only at its posterior and at its right side, and as its left side is almost always bordered by fatty tissue or by connective tissue, connection between the two kinds of muscles takes place only at its posterior end and at its right side. This connection or transition takes place very gradually, so that it is difficult to find a sharp border. Here, the individual small muscle fibers become gradually larger and inconspicuously connect with the ordinary atrial muscle fibers, or else several small muscle fibers in a bundle gradually unite to make a broader muscle fiber, which then enters the ordinary atrial musculature. In the dog, I could not observe the special atrial bundle, running more or less radially in various directions from the posterior end of the connecting bundle and connecting the relatively remote atrial muscle groups with the muscle fibers of the connecting bundle as directly and as straightly as possible. This special atrial bundle might be a so-called mediator, which I described in the case of the sheep heart.

2. *The ventricular segment of the connecting system*

The anterior continuation of the node forms the ventricular segment of the connecting system. As already described, the transition between the atrial and the ventricular segment is relatively gradual. I make the border at the place where the system penetrates the atrioventricular fibrous septum, because this place is easily determined anatomically, and because, at this place in the sheep, the system shows remarkable histological change. I will also divide the ventricular segment into two portions in the dog as in the sheep, i.e. the initial portion, namely from the beginning of the ventricular segment to the upper portion of both the bundle branches and the terminal ramifications.

(a) *The initial portion of the ventricular segment*

The node of the atrial segment gradually becomes smaller when traced forward and continues as the ventricular segment at the entrance of the penetrating canal without undergoing any conspicuous histological change. Only the fiber arrangement becomes more regular than before. After passing obliquely through the base of the aortic wall, the connecting bundle first runs anteriorly for a short distance, separated by aortic tissue on its superior and right sides. On its left side and below, it is also separated by thin connective tissue from the muscular ventricular septum. When the muscle fibers of the initial portion of the ventricular segment are precisely observed, situations similar to those in the node of the atrial segment are found. Here, however, the muscle fibers do not make a complicated network, but show a tendency to run in a more parallel and fascicular arrangement. The individual bundles are separated by abundant connective tissue, and seldom connect with each other. Each bundle is made up of many muscle fibers showing stretched networks. The muscle fibers, therefore, appear to make broad muscle bands with irregularly scattered nuclei. This finding cannot be made in the ordinary cardiac muscle fibers.

When the arrangement of the fibrils is precisely observed, it is seen that the fibrils take on almost the same behavior as that for the node of the atrial segment as described earlier. The fibrils do not run parallel side by side, as in the ordinary ventricular muscle fibers, but are more sparse, look somewhat delicate, and run more or less in a wavy fashion. Both the longitudinal and cross-sectional observations show an irregular arrangement of the fibrils. They are sometimes arranged in relatively broad bundles, but are soon divided into individual fibrils in a fan shape or into many small fibril bundles and, during their further course, join again. In this way, fibrils in the band make an interrelated and longitudinally extended net. Net meshes are thin interfibrillar gaps or relatively wide and clear spindle-shaped or oval fields, in which there is usually a nucleus. When observed more precisely, a border of individual cell territories constituting muscle bands is recognized here and there in the systems of fibrils as longitudinally extended dark borderlines or as real gaps filled with connective tissue. It was not possible crosswise to separate the bands and fibrils with certainty into individual cell territories. I will discuss this issue again in the description of the terminal ramifications of the system. As far as the relation of the amount of fibrils and protoplasm is concerned, it is already well known that the predominance of protoplasm, appearing everywhere as narrow or wide areas between fibril bundles, is observed in longitudinal sections, and much better in cross-sections of the bundles.

At the site of division into the right and left bundle branches, the connecting bundle broadens somewhat. Here, the arrangement of fibrils is still irregular. Fibrils in a muscle fiber run either isolated or in groups of small bundles of fibrils of various sizes, connecting with each other or dividing into numerous individual fibrils. As individual muscle fibers with these fibrils of various arrangements connect with other muscle fibers, the small fibril bundles or individual fibrils continuously run from one muscle fiber into another. In this way, a fibril net is formed which demonstrates the same or similar irregularity as is seen in the plexus at the beginning of the initial portion of the ventricular segment. Here, connective tissue sheaths are similar to those of the beginning of this segment.

Retzer and Humblet, the investigators of the connecting bundle of the dog, described the topography of the bundle only up to the site I just described histologically. Retzer stated definitely that he found no histological differences between this muscular system and the ordinary cardiac musculature other than that the bundle of this system was somewhat looser. Therefore, he thought that there was plenty of connective tissue between the individual muscle fibers of the system. As I already mentioned, I examined many hearts of newborn, young and old dogs and found that there was a considerable histological difference between the bundles of young and adult dogs, but that there was a smaller histological difference among adult dogs. I have never encountered such a case with a histological equality between the fibers of the bundles and the ordinary ventricular musculature such as Retzer reported. The characteristics of the ventricular bundle I described are always found in varying degrees.* In his study of the histology of the bundle performed using an inexpedient method, Humblet reported that the bundle was made up of small interwoven muscle fibers. He did not, however, give any precise description.

In the initial portion of the left and right bundle branches, the histology as a whole is similar to that of the branching site of the bundles. Here, however, muscle complexes are somewhat more simply constructed than those in the upper portion. Individual fibrils of the muscle complexes run more parallel and, over a relatively short course, are not so irregular as in the upper portion.

The muscle complexes here look more longitudinally stretched than in the upper portion (Fig. 1). Gradually, the number of individual muscle fibers running in an orderly fashion increases. In the muscle complexes, thick lines or other similar lines running transversely to the direction of the fibrils, which might represent borders between individual muscle cells, are infrequently recognized. In the fibers running separately, however, the lines were more often recognized. At any rate, cell borders are less frequently seen in this portion than in the terminal ramifications. For example, in heart No. 166, at the beginning of the left bundle branch, I recognized a muscular fiber apparently belonging to the system running about 2.5 mm long without a trace of thick lines or other similar lines indicating cell borders. In this muscle fiber, 12 nuclei lay in succession with various intervals. The histology gradually changes inferiorly. The number of muscle fibers

---

Note at proofreading: According to a kind letter recently received from Prof. Spalteholz, Retzer has also found the structural differences on repeated study of the connecting bundle.

running in a more ordered fashion gradually increases, and the number of fibrils in individual muscle fibers apparently increases. The arrangement of fibrils also becomes more regular than before. This histological change occurs more rapidly in the left bundle branch than in the right. Isolated muscle fibers separated from each other by connective tissue sheaths are soon more predominantly seen in the left bundle branch. On the other hand, in the right bundle branch, this change usually occurs for the first time after the bundle branch passes the place of origin of the several tendinous fibers for the septal leaflet of the tricuspid valve from the ventricular septum, i.e. at the posteroinferior surroundings of the medial papillary muscle. This histological change, nonetheless, occurs so gradually that it is difficult to draw a distinct boundary.

(b) *The lower course of both the bundle branches and the terminal ramifications of the ventricular segment*

In this portion, the muscle fibers of the system as a whole are similar to the ordinary myocardium. When observed precisely, however, small differences are always found. For the purpose of histological study, I made a number of sections and scratch preparations from four hearts of big adult dogs. The findings were relatively different in all hearts. However, they are summarized as follows:

In the dog, the terminal ramifications of the system are never found in the myocardium, but are found exclusively in the subendocardium. The terminal ramifications are more numerous than expected from macroscopical observation. The muscle fibers are usually arranged very loosely, being separated from each other and also from the adjacent ventricular musculature by subendocardial connective tissue fibers or by a laminar connective tissue sheath. Rarely, from the ventricular segment, isolated muscle fibers enter directly the ordinary ventricular muscle fibers. The thickness of the subendocardial connective tissue varies. Muscle fibers are arranged sometimes in one layer, and sometimes in many layers. The direction of individual subendocardial muscle fibers also varies. Sometimes two fibers lying close one upon the other run in entirely different directions, so that cross- or obliquely sectioned fibers are often seen close to a longitudinally sectioned fiber. In the left ventricle the fibers as a whole run in the vertical direction — in other words, parallel to the cardiac axis — while in the right ventricle there is no general direction of the fibers, because the direction is quite different in each portion of the wall.

The individual muscle fibers are always stained somewhat paler than the adjacent ventricular muscle fibers. When observed at stronger magnifications, it is seen that they have other histological peculiarities. In particular, the muscle fibers do not always have straight and parallel borders, as is the case with the ordinary cardiac muscle fibers, but, at certain intervals, they mostly have narrow and slightly constricted sites with bulgy and swollen segments in between. One fiber, therefore, shows alternately narrow and swollen portions in succession. The degree of narrowing varies. It is often only slight, but is sometimes conspicuous (Figs. 2 and 3). The distance from one narrowed site to the next, i.e. the length of individual swollen portions, is relatively equal in one fiber; the length, however, may vary considerably in different fibers. In individual muscle fibers in a bundle, this situation is similar. In muscle fibers in different bundles, however, the situation differs considerably. No narrowed sites are seen in several fibers and, therefore, they have parallel side borders of a considerable length without any narrowing.

When the narrow sites are observed at weaker magnifications, it is first seen that there is not only a side compression but also an overall fiber narrowing represented by broader, usually more or less arched, and dark bands. The bands gradually become obscure in both longitudinal directions of the fiber. At stronger magnifications, it is found that the dark cross-bands are not plain lines but consist of numerous fine fibers closely crowded side by side, running vertically to the lines, i.e. parallel to the direction of the fiber. The fine fibers are cross-striated fibrils mostly running continuously further into the swollen sites. There is no sharp boundary between the cross-band and the muscle fibers of both sides. It is hardly likely that the crowd of the fibrils running parallel onto the band is alone responsible for the dark site. Another special factor for this phenomenon must be searched for, because the dark cross-lines appear at relatively regular intervals. For this purpose, I tried many staining methods and also made scratch preparations. Definite explanation, however, was not obtained.

In scratch preparations, the sites appear as relatively wide and clear cross-bands which, by refracting strong light, usually show no apparent cross- and longitudinal striations. Both the striations appear to originate for the first time at both sides of the cross-bands. When the tube is moved up and down, longitudinal and cross-striations become visible, although faint, also on the clear lines. Furthermore, it is seen that, by moving the tube up and down, the clear cross-bands seldom change their shape and position. It is also seen that, in and along the relatively broad cross-bands, a plain, narrow, more or less curved and fine wavy zigzag line often appears which, according to the height of the tube, looks clear by strong light refraction, or looks dark, or sometimes entirely disappears. I could not make this narrow line more visible in silver staining than in salt solution. When the cross-bands are more precisely examined in sectional preparations, it becomes clear that they are not the same at all sites but show various appearances. Sometimes, the cross-bands show a simple structure. They appear to be constructed of peripheral bundles of fibrils lying more densely in the cross-band than in other parts of the muscle fiber. Here, the axial layer of the fiber shows nothing special. Mostly, however, the cross-bands are constructed in a much more complicated way. When many cross-bands are examined, it is noticed in many instances that the bands are made up of fine fibrils gathered close together, occupying not only the periphery of the band but also all layers of the muscle fiber. In other instances, in the middle of and along the longitudinal direction of the intensively stained cross-bands, a narrow and clear line is shown. The broad and intensively stained bands are separated into two parallel halves by the narrow and clear line, so that it gives an unequivocal impression that here two cells meet at their more or less dull and fitted cell ends (Fig. 3). In these cases, fibrils are always seen to run continuously from one cell to another. Fibrils do not always run perpendicularly on the cross-bands; not infrequently they run obliquely. In addition to the continuous fibrils, new fibrils originate from these sites, i.e. from the side borders of the narrow and clear line, and run irregularly, crossing each other. These fibrils take part in forming the darkly stained bands. From these observations, I consider that the site of narrowing of the muscle fiber, where the fibrils lie densely and irregularly, is the border of the two facing sarcoplasmic territories. I do not intend, however, to imply that there is an actual septum, especially because there is a reliable evidence of continuous transition of certain fibrils. The individual swollen portion of the muscle fiber is, therefore, a sarcoplasmic territory.

Individual sarcoplasmic territories vary in form. Mostly, they are bulgy, somewhat swollen in the middle, and often barrel-shaped or nearly spherical when they are relatively short. There are also sarcoplasmic territories with relatively parallel side borders. The length and width of the sarcoplasmic territories differ. The length is generally three to five times greater than the width. The width is, on the average, much wider than that of the ordinary cardiac musculature. Longitudinal sections show that fibrils are relatively sparse and arranged irregularly. In most of the sarcoplasmic territories, fibrils are arranged near the wall in variously thick layers and run, often arranged as individual or usually as small bundles, from one to another pole of the sarcoplasmic territory. Fibrils do not run as parallel as in the ordinary cardiac muscle fibers, but take a not so orderly course, here and there separating from each other or running obliquely or crossing other fibrils. As illustrated in the cross-section (Fig. 4), the arrangement of fibrils near the wall is not always simple and tubular but is quite varied. Not infrequently, individual fibrils or small groups of fibrils run in various directions inside the cell, connecting and dividing with each other, and form a network extending longitudinally. Sarcoplasm is usually divided by these fibril groups into many, incompletely bordered, each related areas free from fibrils. Rarely, fibrils run in a scattered fashion all through the sarcoplasm, so that there exists no area without fibrils. Bigger fibril-free sarcoplasmic regions show various structures, sometimes fine filament-like, sometimes granular, sometimes vacuolar and sometimes entirely homogeneous. Many of these structures are probably artificial products at the time of fixation. In fresh scratch preparations, usually only nuclei, small fatty corpuscles and at times uncertain granules can be seen in homogeneous sarcoplasm. This condition of sarcoplasm is different from that of the sheep heart, in which, either in the fresh or in the fixed state, rich sarcoplasm is an almost homogeneous and relatively well-stained mass. Probably, sarcoplasm is composed of a relatively watery protein liquid in the dog, whereas the sarcoplasm in the sheep is much more gelatinous.

Nuclei of the muscle fibers of the terminal ramifications do not show a uniform shape. They are, on the average, somewhat shorter, broader and more irregular than those of the ordinary ventricular musculature, in which nuclei are predominantly of an oval or spindle shape. One or two, or seldom three, nuclei are seen in one sarcoplasmic territory. When there are two nuclei, they are either widely separated from each other or lie close side by side or one after the other in the middle of sarcoplasmic territory or in the vicinity of a pole. When there are three nuclei, they are usually arranged in two groups. One nucleus is near a pole, and the other two are close together near another pole. The positional situation, however, is varied.

It is impossible for me to describe all the differences observed in the dog hearts. Nevertheless, I would like to emphasize that the terminal ramifications occasionally show more straightly bordered fibers instead of bulging fibers. In these fibers, the arrangement of fibrils is somewhat more regular. Considerable structural differences exist, nonetheless, between these fibers and the ordinary ventricular muscle fibers. In these fibers, the borderlines of the individual sarcoplasmic territories mentioned earlier often appear distinctly and in a somewhat different form, as indicated in the illustration (Fig. 3). Concerning the question whether these borderlines exist during life and represent actual septation or whether they are just artificial phenomena due to contraction or fixation, I do not intend to answer. I only emphasize that the continuity of fibrils is not interrupted at borderlines, and that the borderlines can be completely absent in scratch preparations of the freshly preserved hearts as well as in several fibers in fixed sectional preparations.

An entirely special histology of this system must be mentioned here. This histology is usually recognized at the sites where the bundle is divided into two or more twigs, or where many bundles coming from different directions meet, connect with each other and form a net. At these sites, the arrangement of the muscle fibers — or, rather, of the fibrils — is very complicated. Individual muscle bundles and muscle fibers are broken up often into many small groups of fibrils or sometimes into individual fibrils. These groups of fibrils or individual fibrils, formerly belonging to a muscle fiber, extend diversely like spread fingers or a fan, and combine with other fibrils originating from other muscle fibers, thus forming a very entangled network, as illustrated schematically in Fig. 9 (scratch preparation).

When such a net is more precisely observed, it is seen that groups of fibrils of various thicknesses run in various planes and in various directions, and cross each other. Individual muscle fibers from different bundles connect with each other in all possible combinations. At the sites of complicated structures, the above-mentioned cross-bands are not infrequently observed. I observed these figures well in the parietal wall of the right ventricle, especially near the anterior papillary muscle. Macroscopically, here, I recognized a very dense subendocardial net formation of the muscle system. These findings are also made at other parts of the wall.

When the essential histological difference between the ordinary cardiac musculature and the muscle fibers of the terminal ramifications of the connecting bundle is briefly summarized, the following must be emphasized: *The muscle fibers of the system are found only in the subendocardium; they are always surrounded by a connective tissue sheath which is much thicker than the perimysium of the cardiac musculature and difficult to scratch off. The muscle fibers consist of numerous relatively short or broad sarcoplasmic territories lying one after another, thus showing distinct border-zones at a certain interval. In the ordinary cardiac muscle fibers of the dog, in contrast, the border-zones are not found, even if contraction lines are observed. Furthermore, the presence of relatively small numbers of fibrils, their irregular course and the accordingly rich sarcoplasm of the terminal ramifications must be enumerated. Finally, highly complicated arrangements of the fibrils at the knotting points of the terminal ramifications are so peculiar that such a figure is never found in the ordinary cardiac musculature.*

In the literature, I found only in Schmalz's work a detailed description concerning the peculiar subendocardial muscle fibers of the dog heart. Although first Aeby, and then Obermeier, saw the peculiar subendocardial muscle fibers, neither gave any precise histological descriptions. In spite of Schmalz's highly appreciated demonstration of Purkinje fibers in the dog, I cannot concur with his interpretations of his figures. He sharply distinguished the cells from the fibril mantle. My study has revealed that such a distinction is impossible. In Purkinje fibers, fibrils are closely connected with sarcoplasm as in other examined animals. The misunderstanding that cells exist separately comes from the fact that, between each sarcoplasmic rich area with nuclei, there are places where only fibrils exist and sarcoplasm is reduced.

I reproduced the figure (Fig. 7) which Schmalz described as Purkinje fibers of the dog heart. Schmalz said that the cells dropped from the fibril nets entangling the cells at the time of scratching. Further, I reproduced another figure (Fig. 8) in which Obermeier described Purkinje fibers of the dog heart. When the figures of these two authors are compared with mine, the difference is very easily seen.

From my investigation of the adult dog heart, it is not possible for me to indicate with certainty that the characteristic cross-bands, especially well recognized in individual muscle fibers of the connecting system of the adult dog heart, are cell borders, although the probability is high that they are cell borders and are not contraction lines like those of the ordinary cardiac musculature. If this problem is to be solved, embryonic or young dog hearts must be investigated. Only in this way can it be decided whether or not Purkinje fibers of the dog heart are truly made up of individual cells which connect secondarily with the fibril system and continue to show their borders.

Unfortunately, for this purpose, only the old sectional preparations of two dogs aged one year were available to me. It became clear from these preparations that the microscopical finding of the terminal ramifications, i.e. Purkinje fibers, is entirely different from that of the adult dog, so that it is hard to believe that the same fiber system is being studied. This is the reason why there is a contradiction among the authors as to the existence or nonexistence of Purkinje fibers in the dog heart (for example, Aeby, Obermeier, Lehnert and so on). Purkinje fibers of the adult dog essentially differ from those of the sheep heart by showing relatively well-developed fibrils and relatively long sarcoplasmic rich extensions, so that only a skillful investigator can recognize the concordance between the two kinds of Purkinje fibers. In fact, the Purkinje fibers of a newborn dog are surprisingly similar to those of an adult sheep. The similarity is the following. The fibers of a newborn dog are also made up predominantly of big, usually oval, protoplasm-rich cell-like structures which are separated from each other by borderlines not only in the longitudinal but also in the cross-direction of the fibers. It must be considered that Purkinje fibers are constructed of solitary elements, in contrast to the ordinary cardiac muscle fibers. Already in a newborn dog, this cell system is intimately connected with a finer system of fibrils running continuously from one cell to the other. Corresponding precisely to the finding on the adult sheep heart, the fibrils first appear at the surface areas of the cells facing each other, but not at the sites where the cells are in contact with a connective tissue sheath (Figs. 5 and 6). It is noteworthy that, in a dog only six days older than the other, the system of fibrils was already much more prominent. In addition to the relatively well-differentiated fibrils, a network of fine fibers, apparently of young fibrils, can barely be recognized in the rich sarcoplasm of individual cells.

It is difficult to answer the question how development of individual cells and their transformation into mature Purkinje fibers proceeds in an adult dog. As individual Purkinje cells not infrequently have two or three nuclei, and as nuclei lie close side by side in a newborn dog but more or less separately in an adult dog, I must make the conclusion that a substantial growth zone does not exist at the so-called cement lines as Heidenhein suggested, but that growth occurs in all cell segments. During the growth of the animals, as fibrils increase, sarcoplasm reduces. Individual sarcoplasmic territories with their nuclei become longer in a longitudinal direction, and sarcoplasm is connected to each other by bridges of fibrillar structures. The cell borders, clearly visible in the young, are now often scarcely or no longer visible, whereas in several fibers they are clearly seen lifelong, as my illustrations (Figs. 2 and 3) show. I can point out the following. Similar cross-lines can also be seen in the ordinary cardiac musculature. However, because of their irregular, often stairlike course, and because of their multiple appearance between two nuclei where there should be only one borderline, and finally because of the situation where they often only partially penetrate the muscle fiber, the cross-lines should be interpreted not as true cement lines, or cell borders, but as dying phenomena of the muscle fibers or so-called contraction lines.

The structural differences of Purkinje fibers emphasized above between newborn and adult dogs are valid also in the atrial segment. In the young dog, the atrial bundle is composed of big cells, in contrast to fiber-shaped cells in the adult dog.

(c) *Human heart*

The course and extent of the atrioventricular connecting bundle in the human heart have already been discussed precisely in the anatomical chapter. If I describe the histology in detail, I must repeat what I have mentioned

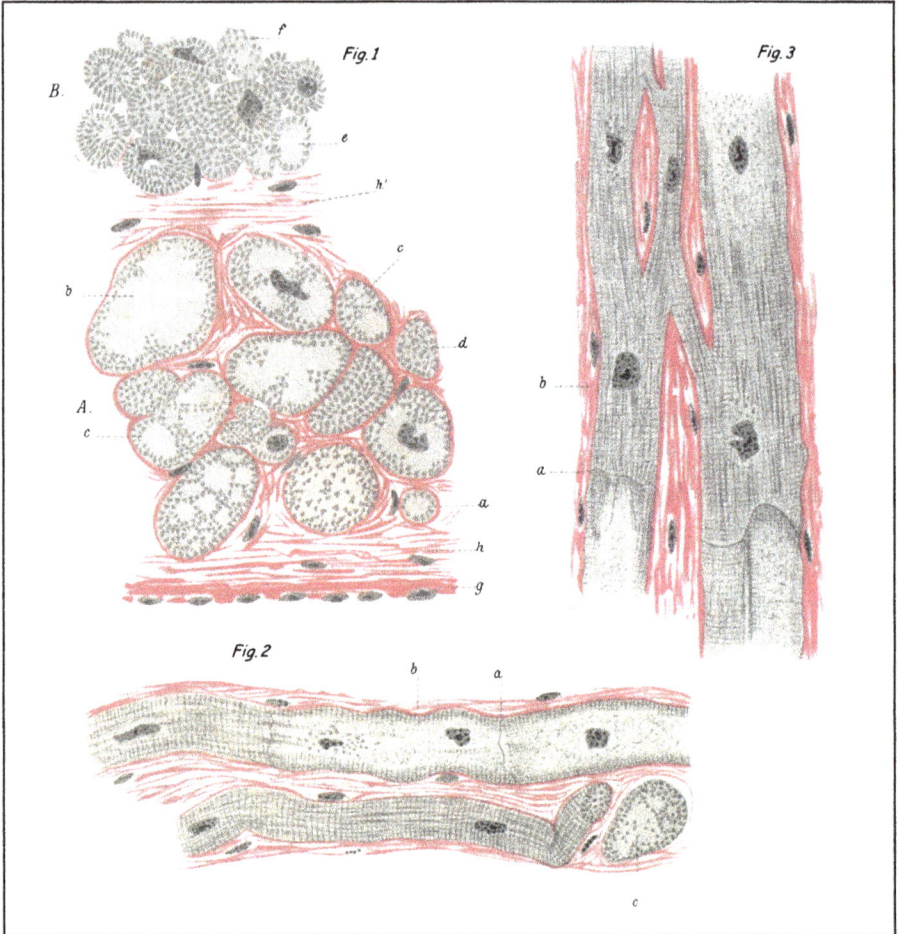

Histology of the atrioventricular connecting system of the human heart

Fig. 1. Cross-section of muscle fibers of the terminal ramification of the ventricular connecting bundle. It can be seen that the thickness of individual fibers varies conspicuously. The fibril arrangement also varies.

A = group of muscle fibers of the ventricular bundle

a = a thin muscle fiber with one-layer fibril mantle

b = a very thick fiber with peripheral fibril layers

c = partition of sarcoplasm into fields by fibril bundles

d = a fiber with scattered fibrils

B = ordinary ventricular muscle fibers with fibrils which are schematically illustrated (see text, pp. 153–154)

$e \& f$ = ordinary ventricular muscle fibers with a peripheral fibril mantle and with scattered thin fibrils respectively (see text, p. 154)

g = endocardium

h = subendocardial connective tissue

h' = subendocardial connective tissue which separates the ventricular bundle of the connecting system from the ordinary ventricular musculature

Figs. 2 & 3. Longitudinal section of muscle fibers of the terminal ramification of the ventricular bundle, i.e. human Purkinje fibers

a = probably a cell border

b = subendocardial connective tissue

c = a cross-sectioned Purkinje fiber

about the dog heart, because there are many similarities between the findings observed in the human and in the dog. It is of great significance, therefore, when one utilizes the facts obtained in the dog experiments.

Here, only several small differences will be described between the fibers of the atrioventricular connecting bundle and the terminal ramifications in the dog and the human. The atrial segment of the bundle in the human is constituted not of densely pressed and partially fused fibers, as is often the case in the dog, but mostly of a network made up of well traceable and thin individual fibers, as seen in the other animals. The extent of the formation of nets in the human heart is relatively small, although it varies in cases. The initial portion of the ventricular bundle in the human is exclusively constituted of individual fibers running in a parallel fashion, whereas in the dog a unique fusion of the fibers is seen. *Individual muscle fibers of the terminal ramifications in the human seem to possess, on the average, more fibrils than in the dog and, therefore, resemble more the ordinary ventricular muscle fibers.*

Several other peculiarities found in the fibers of the human connecting bundle are usually ascribed to pathological processes of the hearts examined. These differences are also observed well in the terminal ramifications, i.e. the human Purkinje fibers.

As to the evidence of essential concordance between the human and the dog, several illustrations of the fibers of the terminal ramifications of the human heart (Figs. 1–3) will be shown. I tried to reproduce as naturally as possible the characteristic arrangement of fibrils. Also here, as in the dog heart, predominance of sarcoplasm over fibrils is clearly noted. Fibrils, illustrated as small triangles, are arranged more peripherally and irregularly (Fig. 1). Here, I should emphasize that the triangle is chosen arbitrarily and that there are, in fact, many variations in cross-sectional figures of the individual fibril bundles. I could not reproduce individual variations in the illustrations, because it was more important for me to show the characteristic position of the fibrils in the fibers. I described the situation in the dog heart in detail, how sarcoplasm predominates over fibrils in the whole fiber system of the atrioventricular connecting bundle, and how fibrils gradually increase in number in the terminal ramifications, with the arrangement becoming much more similar to that of the ordinary cardiac muscle fibers, consequently resulting in difficulty in finding any difference between the two systems. All my descriptions of the dog heart are also observed in the human heart.

Here, it should be mentioned that also in the ordinary ventricular musculature there are rarely fibers which, as with those of the terminal ramifications, show abundant sarcoplasm outside of the nucleus, and have a more annular arrangement of bundles of fibrils in the periphery or irregularly scattered sparse fibrils in the sarcoplasm (Fig. 1, *e, f*). Because I found these fibers only in the hearts, especially in the heart of a patient dying from cancer cachexia, a pathological process of the fibers must be considered.

Here, I will refer to the remark appearing in Kölliker's textbook[12] that in cross-section the bundles of fibrils in the periphery of the fibers show a band form. Although I fairly frequently found the structure described by this author in the dog, I did not find it in the human. I cannot confirm, therefore, the structure as characteristic for the fibers of the human heart. Also, the generally accepted view that sarcoplasm spreads in the form of a radially arranged network from the center of a fiber to its periphery is not consistent with my findings. Rather, the network is constructed of irregular meshes usually made up of fine sarcoplasmic networks. Of course, the findings are remarkable in Purkinje fibers. Those who are not acquainted with the coarse sarcoplasmic networks in normal Purkinje fibers may easily mistake them as pathological products. The figures described by Albrecht[2] (in his Plate VI, Fig. 12) as pathological are found everywhere in normal Purkinje fibers.

Another histological peculiarity of the terminal ramifications is that the entire volume of individual fibers, as well as of nuclei, although the volumes exceed or are equal to those in the ordinary ventricular muscle fibers, remain behind the volumes of the ventricular muscle fibers in the setting of considerable hypertrophy of the ventricular muscle. This is because, in such cases, the muscle fibers of the connecting bundle seem to take little, if any, part in the hypertrophy. Inversely, in advanced atrophy, the volumes of the connecting bundle exceed those of the ordinary cardiac muscle fibers.

Strong pigmentation, frequently found in the nuclear region of the ordinary human cardiac muscle fibers, also appears to a limited extent in the fibers of the ventricular bundle of the connecting system.

The following might be the most important peculiarities to be emphasized in the system of the human atrioventricular connecting bundle. Unfortunately for me, it was not possible to make a definite conclusion on the question whether or not there are true cell borders, i.e. transverse partitions in the fibers of the human terminal ramifications. Even though, by examining numerous preparations of the ordinary cardiac musculature, I am convinced that all that were described as cement lines or cell borders showed no positive evidences for cell borders, and that they must rather be considered as abnormally contracting or dying phenomena, I am inclined to admit to the existence of cell borders, at least in many fibers of the ventricular bundle of the connecting system. It is possible, nonetheless, that even these apparent cell borders are only artificial products. In various characteristics, however, they are different from the well-known cement lines of the ordinary cardiac muscle fibers. The characteristics are as follows:

(1) When the muscle fibers of the terminal ramifications are followed longitudinally, peculiar cross-bands are recognized in many fibers. Finer structures of the bands could not be precisely investigated.

(2) The cross-bands are often well visible at the axial site of the fiber where there exists only sarcoplasm and no fibrils are developed. The bands, therefore, cannot be abnormal contractions of the fibrils.

(3) Several fibrils appear to end just at this site, although most of the fibrils run without interruption.

(4) The cross-bands never lie in the nuclear territory but between the two nuclei.

(5) The cross-bands are neither formed in a stair shape nor arranged in two or more lines running close together or parallel, as is often the case with the so-called cement lines in the ordinary cardiac muscle fibers; but the bands are always visible as arched or wavy lines on the entire fiber breadth at a certain distance.

(6) In van Gieson preparations, the bands are stained neither like fibrils nor like protoplasm, but stained somewhat reddish and like connective tissue.

(7) The muscle fibers are often strangulated at the sites where cross-bands are visible, although not so markedly as seen in the dog heart.

(8) The cross-bands are mostly thin and usually sharply separated from the adjacent sarcoplasm. The cross-band is not a connective tissue fiber which runs above or beneath the muscle fiber or twists around it or constricts it. This can be confirmed by the different staining behavior as well as by the configuration of the entire fiber obtained through careful use of the fine focus adjustment of the microscope.

(9) I have many preparations in which cross-bands are clearly visible in the muscle fibers of the connecting bundle, whereas there are no cross-bands in the ordinary cardiac muscle fibers. At any rate, these findings indicate that the connecting muscle fibers must be morphologically constructed differently from the ordinary cardiac muscle fibers. Otherwise, the differences between the two kinds of muscle in the same preparation are not explicable.

My attempt to demonstrate, using the embryonic hearts kindly offered to me by Professor Gasser and the eight fetal hearts prepared in serial sections, the gradual development of the connecting system and its composition from isolated cells or continuous fibers failed, because they were not preserved in the way of answering the question. I was not able to prepare new material. It was extraordinarily difficult to demonstrate the course and direction of individual fibers or cells of the system in each or in serial sections, because of the underdevelopment of the fibrils, the smallness of the object, and the complicated structure of the atrioventricular connecting bundle. I can hardly say, therefore, whether apparently visible cell borders are indicative of just oblique or cross-sectional lines of the fibers or of the true borders of round or oval cells. I generally have an impression, nonetheless, that, in the atrial segment of the human heart, the demarcation of individual cells probably occurs at an early stage or until the end of the fetal development. On the other hand, in contrast to the dog, the ventricular bundle of the human shows a structure of unusually long and unsegmented fibers by the late months of fetal life.

As the proof of this assumption, I will briefly describe the histological findings on several human fetal hearts. In the 10- to 11-week-old embryonic heart (No. 170), the atrial segment of the connecting system is already well recognized. At weak magnification, it apparently looks paler than the ordinary cardiac musculature. At stronger magnification, it is seen that the atrial segment is composed of conspicuously pale and relatively large cells. The cells lie close side by side, or one upon the other, and appear to have mostly an irregularly round form. Most of the nuclei are regularly round or oval. The cell body is so transparent that, in most of the cells, almost nothing can be seen except for a relatively large vesicular nucleus. In several cells, however, a small number of fine fibrils, or seldom a complicated fibrillar network, can be seen. Besides these extraordinarily fine fibrils with barely visible striations, coarser cross-striated fibrils can be sparsely seen, running continuously from one cell to the other. When these findings are compared with those on the ordinary atrial musculature in the same heart, a considerable difference is already recognizable at this stage. The ordinary atrial musculature already shows muscle fibers with a delicate and monolayered fibril mantle in their peripheries. In the ventricle, only the upper portion of the left bundle branch was convincingly identified. It appeared to be made up of large cells with more fibrils than the atrial segment, but less fibrils than the ordinary ventricular muscle fibers. It is separated from the ventricular musculature by thin connective tissue. I could not confirm in these serial sections whether or not the individual cells were the cross- or oblique sectional surfaces of the individual muscle fibers.

In the approximately 17-week-old embryonic heart (No. 172), fibrils in the atrial segment have already developed to some extent, but they are recognized at several sites only as relatively narrow and short small bundles or as individual fibrils. Therefore, one cannot yet recognize completely differentiated muscle fibers. At this embryonic stage, as far as could be concluded from the stained sections, the atrial segment appears to be made up mostly of vesicular and oval cells connecting one after the other and fusing. In the ventricular septum, both of the bundle branches can be seen in their typical sites. The bundle branches already appear to consist mostly of long muscle fibers — with fibrils, however, which are still delicate and sparsely developed. Both of the bundle branches are separated from the ordinary cardiac musculature by thin but highly recognizable connective tissue fibers. Terminal ramifications of both the bundle branches were recognized with difficulty, because there were no characteristics worth mentioning except for poor development of fibrils and, on the average, larger thickness of the individual cells to differentiate them from the ordinary ventricular muscle fibers. The ordinary cardiac musculature already consists of highly traceable muscle fibers connecting with each other. At the peripheries, the fibers usually have a layer of relatively well-developed fibrils.

In the heart of a seven-month-old premature baby (No. 162), differentiation of crosswise and longitudinally striated muscle fibers of the system has developed to a stage where the atrial segment consists of long and thin muscle fibers, connecting with each other and forming a characteristic network.

During the further course of fetal and extrauterine life, as the heart grows, the fibrils increase in number in the muscle fibers of the connecting bundle as well as in the ordinary cardiac musculature, and finally reach the adult condition at 12–15 years of life.

I will not discuss the questions as to from which embryonic layer the system originates, and in which embryonic week the system is ready for the entire development. It is undoubtedly accepted, however, that in the human heart, in the first two to three embryonic weeks, the system is unable to exist as in the adult heart, because the ventricular septum does not exist at this stage.

Finally, a question arises whether Purkinje fibers of the human I described have already been observed by other authors. The only statement under this consideration appears in Kölliker's textbook. It says, "In the human, Purkinje fibers never exist regularly... *[p. 618]*. In the ventricular musculature of the human being, just beneath the endocardium, there exist fibers representing a duct consisted of cross-straited fibrils *[p. 607, left, Fig. 1257]*. The hollow space is enlarged, filled with sarcoplasm and a nucleus. There is a constriction between the enlarged portions. The fibrils approach each other at the constriction, resulting in disappearance of the brightness of the duct. Further, during their long course, the ducts lying side by side fuse together with their fibril mantles. As a result, a transitional form between the cardiac muscle fibers and Purkinje cells is actually formed *[p. 626]*." This description is applicable only to a part of Purkinje fibers of the human according to my description. The majority of the fibrils demonstrate neither constrictions nor regular ductal arrangement. Probably, as Kölliker, based upon the findings on the sheep heart, looked for such fibers and found an equivalent of Purkinje fiber of the sheep heart, he must never have thought of any relationship between the peculiar fibers and the atrioventricular connecting system, and of the concordance of the system with that of Purkinje fibers of the sheep heart.

In addition to the hearts of the human and other animals described before, I examined the hearts of rabbits, rats, guinea pigs, and a pigeon heart among the birds. The results of the examinations are briefly presented here.

(d) *Rabbit heart*

I did not examine this heart macroscopically. In the serial sectional preparations, I confirmed that the atrial segment of the atrioventricular connecting bundle consisted of crowded net-forming muscle fibers characterized by abundant nuclei. As the ventricular segment exhibits no apparent histological differences from the ordinary ventricular muscle fibers, I could only partially trace the course through serial examination.

(e) *Rat heart*

I also examined this heart serially. The result, however, was by no means satisfactory because of the smallness of the muscle fibers. I was able to differentiate with certainty only the atrial segment and the initial portion of the ventricular bundle from the ordinary cardiac musculature. Also in the rat heart, the atrial segment of the bundle demonstrated a complicated network of fibers. As the ventricular bundle consisted of the muscle fibers difficult to be differentiated from the fibers of the ordinary ventricular musculature, I could not trace with certainty each of the terminal ramifications.

(f) *Guinea pig heart*

I examined one guinea pig heart macroscopically. Although at a glance I recognized no terminal ramifications in the subendocardium, there were numerous fine tendinous fiber-like cords of wool hair thickness in the ventricle. The cords distinctly formed a network in the left ventricle as in the cat heart.

Microscopically, I examined only a part of the ventricular septum where the left bundle branch was thought to run, and I found it there. The left bundle branch was found in the subendocardium, and it consisted of relatively thick and pale muscle fibers with only a small number of fibrils. The muscle fibers of the subendocardial terminal ramifications, as well as of the tendinous fiber-like cords I described macroscopically earlier, demonstrated no great difference from those of the ordinary ventricular muscle fibers. The muscle fibers of the connecting bundle, however, had distinct interstitial connective tissue or connective tissue sheaths for individual muscle fibers. The fibers exhibited cross- or longitudinal striations more obscurely than the ordinary ventricular fibers.

(g) *Pigeon heart*

This heart was also examined in serial sections. As the sectional direction was not correct, I was unable to trace the entire course of the connecting bundle. The pigeon heart surely possesses an atrioventricular connecting bundle. Together with Obermeier and Hofmann, I also found Purkinje fibers in the pigeon heart. Histologically, Purkinje fibers consisted of thick fibers containing relatively sparse and especially delicate fibrils and weakly stained, large and mostly round nuclei. The cell bodies are conspicuously transparent. Not infrequently, Purkinje fibers appear to be constructed of short cells connected one after the other. On the other hand, there are also fibers showing no cell borders for a long distance. The terminal ramifications are mostly found in the subendocardium. As already observed by Hofmann, however, the fibers often take a course into deeper layers accompanied by larger myocardial branches of arteries. Transitions from the peculiar fibers to the ordinary cardiac muscle fibers are frequently seen. The transitions have no special characteristics.

C. Critical Review and Conclusion

The essential result of my study provides evidence of the regularity of the course and the characteristic structure of the connecting bundle in all the hearts of mammalian animals examined, which distinguishes the connecting bundle from the ordinary cardiac musculature. The characteristic structure is especially distinctive in the hearts of ungulates. I believe that I have offered the proof that Purkinje fibers are no more than the terminal ramifications of the connecting bundle between the atrial and the ventricular musculature. The significance of these Purkinje fibers has not been explained until now.

Now that the physiological significance of Purkinje fibers is held to be the same as that of the atrioventricular bundle, I think it important to make once again a historical review of this matter, and also to make a critical review concerning the extent to which Purkinje fibers have already been proved to exist in mammalian animals other than ungulates before my study, and concerning what physiological significance has been given to Purkinje fibers.

I. Development of the Theories on Purkinje Fibers

In 1845, Purkinje[13] discovered a net of gray, flat and gelatinous fibers under the serous membrane of the inner wall of the ventricles of the sheep heart. He found microscopically that the fibers were composed of numerous corns* with nuclei, and that the corns gathered tightly in a polyhedral form. "In each corn, there are one or two nuclei without spherical surrounding as usually seen in the ganglion corns. Five to ten of the corns exist in the transverse direction, and the corns are also arranged in the vertical direction in rows in a bundle. Thus, these corns make up the gray fibers. Between the corns in the stroma of the ventricular walls, there exists an elastic tissue of double fibers which shows cross-striations, when treated by vinegar, like in the ordinary cardiac muscle fibers." Purkinje was not able, however, to decide whether the fibers were actually muscle fibers or just a contour of the membranous walls which surrounded the content of the corns as in plant cells.

Concerning the significance of this peculiar structure, Purkinje was first inclined to consider it something like cartilaginous tissue. But its significance was not clear for him. It was more probable to him that the structure had something to do with a special motor apparatus, and he thought that the membrane surrounding the corns was muscular.

He also discovered similar corn fibers in the cow, pig and horse, but he was not successful in finding the fibers in the human, dog, rabbit and hare.

In 1852, in his *Handbook of Histology*, v. Kölliker[14] described the result of his study of Purkinje fibers as follows: "These fibers are composed of large and polygonal cells with beautiful nuclei, and probably contain a cross-striated mass only at their wall. The cells are unable to be differentiated from cardiac muscle fibers." v. Kölliker claimed to have observed microscopically the contraction of the fibers in the fresh endocardium of the bovine. For these reasons, he considered the fibers to be muscle tissue.

Later, v. Kölliker described the function of Purkinje fibers as follows: "The fibers present an embryonic form and, with regard to the size of the cells, a peculiarly developed form of cardiac muscle fibers. The fibers show manifold transition to the ordinary cardiac muscle fibers by cell fusing."

In 1854, Theodor v. Heßling[15] published his detailed study of Purkinje fibers in the sheep, pig, calf and goat. According to him, Purkinje fibers formed diverse nets and meshes in the subendocardium in the ruminants, which constantly appeared more dominantly in the left than in the right ventricle. Usually, the fibers combined widely together, forming a

---

*Korn

membranous plate, in which only a few small gaps were seen (in the sheep). According to him, Purkinje fibers were found not only in the subendocardial or intramuscular layer, but also, not infrequently, in the subpericardium. Mostly, the fibers were lost in the muscular substance; at times they gradually became thinner in width, finishing with their dull endings. The corns were a solid substance of wax consistency and showed marked transparency. They had one to three nuclei and were usually striated into several directions. He mentioned that Purkinje fibers were made up of several corns lying side by side and one after the other, and of a sheath holding them together which had a property of the cardiac muscle fiber.

As to the significance of Purkinje fibers, his opinion was not conclusive: "... it seems to me that the corns are nothing but pieces of separated muscle substance lying side by side, which appear too constantly to be regarded as pathological." His study of the heart of the roebuck supported his opinion and he mentioned: "These corns are pieces of decomposed muscle cords or bundles in the ordinary cardiac muscle tissue; their appearance, especially in the ruminants, has no physiological significance."

C. B. Reichert[16] quoted v. Heßling's study in his article "Advancement in Microscopical Anatomy in the Year of 1854." Concerning the corns, he endorsed v. Heßling's findings in general. He objected, however, to v. Heßling's opinion that Purkinje fibers were composed of corns and ordinary cardiac muscle substance between the corns. Reichert considered the striations as crosswise or longitudinally shining side walls of the corns. He also considered that the sheath embedding Purkinje fibers was made up of connective tissue.

Concerning the significance of Purkinje fibers, Reichert took the view that these structures were nothing but cross-striated ordinary cardiac muscle fibers, or primitive muscle cylinders which were extraordinarily short, thick and transparent, and were provided in their axis by the nuclei and granular mass which frequently appeared in embryonic, cross-striated muscle fibers. According to him, the short muscle cylinders were directed with their blunt ends toward the ordinary cardiac muscle mass, and with their opposite ends toward the endocardial elastic fiber layer. Taking their location into account, he considered that the short primitive muscle bundles must stretch the endocardium and its tendon-like branches at the time of contraction. He supposed that the structure was a netlike spread stretching muscle of the endocardium — in other words, a tensor of the endocardium — and that the primitive muscle bundles behaved differently from the ordinary cardiac musculature.

In 1862 there appeared the study of Remak[17]: "Embryological Basis of Cytology." He described Purkinje fibers of the sheep and cow hearts as cross-striated and anastomosing cardiac muscle fibers interrupted here and there by "large gelatinous balls." Obviously for him, this arrangement has the purpose of reducing as far as necessary the contraction of the cardiac muscle fibers in the firm and elastic endocardium in order to prevent complete emptying of the cardiac chambers. It appeared to him that complete emptying did not occur in these animals, as proved by opening the transversely sectioned hearts after death.

In 1863, Ch. Aeby[18] published his study of Purkinje fibers. Regarding the morphological aspects, he essentially confirmed v. Heßling's statements. According to him, Purkinje fibers were found predominantly under the endocardium, and rarely in the ventricular wall. Generally, the cells were arranged in a cordlike or sheetlike fashion. Where two cells met, instead of a simple line, a rosary figure was often seen, which, he thought, was due to empty spaces or vacuoles. There were also longer cells like a pumpkin seed, and the fibers made up of such cells often resembled tapeworms. He objected, however, to v. Heßling's opinion that the corns were connected by a cement substance having the characteristics of the cardiac muscle fiber. Like v. Kölliker, he believed that the striped mass was a part of the cell, and that it frequently took on the form of a peripheral mantle.

Aeby considered Purkinje fibers as forms developing into the ordinary cardiac muscle fibers. Indeed, he insisted that the cardiac muscle fibers of all animals originated from Purkinje cells, which became cylindrical fibers by fusing with each other. As evidence, he referred to the occasional appearance of the partitions in the ordinary cardiac muscle fibers, which, he insisted, were found in all hearts of the humans and other animals. From his viewpoint, these partitions were rests of the membranes of individual Purkinje cells remaining as a result of incomplete fusion. In the human and other animals in which he could not find Purkinje cells, all the developing materials were supposed by him to have already been consumed in the early stage. Transformation into the ordinary cardiac muscle fibers, he thought, occurred during a long period, or even continued throughout life. Purkinje fibers were exactly the cells giving rise to the cardiac muscle fibers. He admitted to the possibility of continuing regular production of new muscle fibers in older age, because fusion of the cells was still observed in older age.

Apart from the ruminants, Aeby found Purkinje fibers in the dog, cat, Mustela foina and hedgehog, as well as in the chicken of at least nearly adult stage. In contrast, he confirmed that Purkinje fibers were absent in the human and rabbit, as well as in the house mouse and mole.

C. J. Eberth[19] histologically examined in detail the structure of the cardiac muscle of the human, various animals and birds using silver staining or isolation of individual fibers by a 35% potassium solution or various combined methods. He published in 1866 his work, "Concerning Elements of the Cross-striated Muscle." Here, he thought he had demonstrated that the heart was composed of short or long muscle cells with one or more nuclei. He rejected the fusing phenomenon of muscle cells. According to him, the size and form of the cellular elements varied considerably, and the elements were connected by cement substance. He did not differentiate Purkinje cells from the ordinary cardiac cells, but rather described Purkinje cells as short elements of the cardiac muscle with many nuclei. These short muscle cells, connected by cement substance, formed netlike branching cords under the endocardium and lay "as gap-filling mass in cement substance like wall stones in mortar." He made no mention of the physiological significance of the cells.

In the following year, Obermeier[20] gave a comprehensive description of the fibers in his work, "Structure and Texture of Purkinje Fibers." Concerning their form and characteristic brightness, he compared the fibers with cell cartilage of various fishes. When the fibers were freshly curetted, long and slender polyhedral bodies usually dropped out. Like v. Heßling, he named them "corns." The corns had an oval cylindrical form, and a smooth or somewhat folded surface. He denied the presence of the intervening substance described by v. Heßling, and never saw fibrils falling down from the corns, or decomposition of the corns. His definition of Purkinje corns was as follows: cylindrical or oval bodies with hyalinous axis substance in which nuclei and so on were embedded, and with longitudinally or crosswise striated peripheral substance. He also emphasized the connective tissue sheath of Purkinje fibers. He classified the corns into three different types:

(1)   Highly transparent and shining corns without sharp markings which indicate longitudinal or cross-striations.

(2)   Corns showing less transparency but distinct longitudinal or cross-striations. They are generally slender in shape. Cross-sectional observation shows less hyalinous mass than for cross-striated substance.

(3)   Corns similar to the cross-striated muscle fiber, and generally slender and longer than the other Purkinje corns. In these, hyalinous mass is observed to some extent.

Further, Obermeier precisely described how, at many sites, the corns gradually became slender and longer, and were provided by cross- or longitudinal striations becoming like primitive cardiac muscle bundles; in other words, how they connected with the ordinary cardiac muscle fibers. Obermeier considered, nonetheless, that the cardiac muscle fibers were not fully demonstrated to develop from Purkinje fibers. Rather, he considered, "It is natural to think that Purkinje fibers provide, through their peculiar netlike arrangement, better tightening of the endocardium during cardiac contraction." He insisted that he had found, through his precise comparative study, that the endocardial elastic fiber layer was more strongly developed in the animals in which no Purkinje fibers were found.

Obermeier found Purkinje fibers in the sheep, cow, pig, horse, dog, goose and pigeon. He did not find them in the cat, human, hare, mouse and frog.

In 1868, Max Lehnert[21] published his comprehensive study, "Concerning Purkinje Fibers," in *Archives of Microscopical Anatomy*. He constantly found Purkinje fibers in the calf, sheep, cow, pig, horse, deer and goat. He tried in vain to find them in the human, dog, hare, rabbit, fox, mole, cat, rat, mouse, heron, goose, chicken, pigeon, siskin, frog, and in the carp and pike among fishes. From his viewpoint that Purkinje fibers must contain individual corns separable from each other, he did not agree with Obermeier's view that the fibers he found in the dog, chicken, pigeon and goose were Purkinje cells.

Lehnert understood Purkinje fibers as those composed of numerous, netlike arranged and manifoldly crossing and intervening pieces of cross-striated muscle fibrils, with meshes which were filled with Purkinje corns. He thought that the corns were nothing but meaningless remnants of hyalinous material used originally to make the substance of Purkinje fibers. He differentiated central fibrils from peripheral fibrils. He believed that the central fibrils originated from peripheral fibrils entering the corns, taking their courses in certain or uncertain directions and often forming an entangled fibril cluster in the corns. He supposed that fibrils of Purkinje fibers branched from the ordinary cardiac muscle bundles and, having formed meshes for the corns in Purkinje fibers, again ran further as the ordinary muscle bundles. All in all, he considered that Purkinje fibers were only a peculiar phenomenon along the course of certain myocardial fibril bundles, appearing in a small number of mammalian animals, and that it was difficult to interpret Purkinje fibers as a special and independent organ. He felt, judging from the peculiar courses of fibrils, that those authors admitting the cellular construction of Purkinje fibers were misled.

From Lehnert's standpoint, therefore, Purkinje fibers have no physiological significance other than that of representing the ordinary cardiac muscle fibers arranged as a net.

In the study of Anton Frisch[22] (1869), I found the following statements. Purkinje fibers appear only in the hearts of several mammalian animals (sheep, goat, deer, cow, horse and pig). He definitely rejected Obermeier's statement that Purkinje fibers exist in the hearts of the dog, goose, chicken and pigeon. He did not recognize Purkinje fibers in the hearts of the headgehog and marten, in which Aeby saw the fibers. He considered Henle's description untrue that Purkinje fibers appear in the hearts of the newborn baby. He did not find either the fibers in the heart of the eagle and of *spermophilus citillus*.

Frisch noticed that, in the left ventricle, Purkinje fibers made a regularly formed net as high as the level of the papillary muscles, whereas the fibers became scattered without apparent net formation above the level of the papillary muscles. He also stated that a strong bundle of Purkinje fibers made by combination of two separate cords coming from the papillary muscles went toward the arterial orifice, gradually became unclear, and disappeared several millimeters below the origin of the aorta. According to him, Purkinje fibers of this strong cord connected here with the fibers of ordinary muscular substance.

A fully developed Purkinje fiber was described to be composed microscopically of polygonal, clear and gelatinous cells having one or two round nuclei, and being separated from each other by fibrils of a cross-striated muscular substance. These large cells, the corns of a Purkinje fiber, were embedded in a fiberwork of muscle fibrils, from which the fibrils passed through the corns. Like v. Heßling and Lehnert, therefore, he accepted two special components in Purkinje fibers: corns and cross-striated muscle fibrils.

In addition, Frisch studied Purkinje fibers of the sheep and pig embryos. According to him, already in the 6–9-centimeter-long embryo, a delicate net of corn-shaped protoplasmic cords with numerously scattered nuclei was found under the endocardium. Polygonal and flat cells with beautiful nuclei appeared clearly in this delicate net of corn-shaped protoplasm. The cells gradually became larger and, in later stages, showed longitudinal and cross-striations first arising at the margin. Now followed the stage where cross-striation spread all over the cells. Then individual corns began to swell uniformly. The cross-striated substance formed a thin layer at the superior and inferior surfaces of the corns, and fibrils appeared more thickly and numerously at the sides than in the inner substance. This was the completely developed stage of Purkinje fibers.

On the function of Purkinje fibers, Frisch did not say anything certain. He did not agree with any of the hypotheses proposed by many authors, but concluded his study with the following remark: "In spite of all, however, we must think over the question as to by what the mechanics of the hearts with and without Purkinje fibers is differentiated."

F. Schweigger-Seidel made the following description of Purkinje fibers in *Stricker's Handbook of the Human and Animal Histology*, which was published in 1871: "The ventricular endocardium has all vascular wall layers, and not only intima but all the other vascular layers can be identified." He also supposed that muscular tissue participated in constructing the ventricular endocardium in the form of smooth as well as cross-striated fibers. Concerning cross-striated fibers, he stated that they appeared in two forms: as the well-known Purkinje fibers and as a large meshed net of muscle bundles which were, at best, distinguished from the ordinary cardiac muscle fibers by their size (broader width and shorter longitudinal diameter). He also stated that each Purkinje fiber was composed of more or less regular and prismlike corns; each corn was composed of cross-striated fibrillary muscle substance in the periphery and hyalinous substance with one or two clear nuclei in the axis. He considered each corn as a muscle cell in which (like in the embryonic stage) only the peripheral layer was converted into contractile substance. He thought that the controversy on the existence of Purkinje fibers in this or that animal had little meaning, because it was only a matter of variance of endocardial muscle. According to him, the important point was to explain precisely the developmental history concerning the relation of Purkinje fibers to the cardiac muscles in the developed stage. He expressed nothing about the significance of Purkinje fibers.

In the textbook *General and Microscopical Anatomy* by Krause, which appeared in 1876, there is also a short remark on Purkinje fibers. Krause wrote particularly that "They are secondary muscle bundles of a series of polyhedral contractile muscle cells staying on the embryonic stage. The cells are cross-striated only in the periphery. In the axis with nuclei, differentiation of contractile protoplasm into anisotropic and isotropic substance either does not occur at all, or only in the form of scattered small pieces of muscle." He did not find Purkinje fibers in the human, rabbit and so on.

In the same year, Henle wrote in his *Handbook of Human Angiology* (p. 63) concerning Purkinje fibers as follows: In the first month of life of the human, and in the adult stage of various animals, gray fiber nets of cells, standing side by side, with the shape of a pumpkin seed, appear under the endocardium. The cells show transitions in various ways to cross-striated muscle bundles and actually seem to be a new layer of membrane engaging in construction of the cardiac wall.

Henle claimed that he had found the peculiar Purkinje fibers in a very young human, while all other investigators thus far did not find Purkinje fibers in the human.

In his *Technical Textbook of Histology*, translated into German in 1877, L. Ranvier discussed in detail Purkinje fibers. According to him, Purkinje cells forming a Purkinje fiber showed longitudinal and cross-striation at the margins of a corn-shaped protoplasmic mass containing one or usually two oval nuclei at the center. The thickness of the striated layer was smaller at the free surface than at the surface facing the neighboring cells. It seemed as if the cells were surrounded by a net of muscle fibers. There were longitudinal and cross-striations on the free surface which seemed to belong to the cells. Using a 40% potassium solution, Ranvier disintegrated the fibers into individual cells and, in these free cells, he demonstrated fibrillary striation. Supported by this fact, he definitely rejected Lehnert's view that the striated peripheral substance was an independent muscular net in which Purkinje cells were simply enclosed. He stated also that he had confirmed the transition of Purkinje fibers to the cardiac muscle fibers.

Ranvier considered, like many other authors, Purkinje fibers to be embryonic cardiac muscle fibers arrested in their development.

In 1877, Gegenbauer[23] reported that he had observed the appearance of Purkinje fibers in a 15-year-old human at many sites in the right ventricular myocardium. The structure was almost the same as that of Purkinje fibers of the sheep. He regarded the fibers as cardiac muscle elements having developed in a peculiar direction, and not as muscle cells simply staying in their development. According to him, the peripheral layer of the contractile substance of the fibers was altered, compressed by enlargement of the undifferentiated cell substance, to a thin layer interrupted here and there by wide gaps. On the other hand, in the ordinary cardiac fibers, the undifferentiated cell substance gradually reduced in proportion to differentiation of the contractile peripheral layer. He said nothing about the physiological significance of Purkinje fibers.

In 1886, R. Schmaltz[24] reported in detail on this subject in his study, "Purkinje Fibers in the Heart of Domestic Mammalian Animals." He found Purkinje fibers of the horse heart as the most suitable object for investigation. Starting with this animal, he studied precisely and compared the fibers in the goat, cow, sheep and pig. He found some difference between the animal species, and, especially in the dog and rabbit, he confirmed considerable differences in comparison with the above-mentioned ungulates. Schmaltz found Purkinje fibers in almost all the domestic mammalian animals, and considered this point especially important. He did not study the human heart. He presumed, however, the existence of Purkinje fibers also in the human.

From the viewpoint of developmental history, Schmaltz also studied Purkinje fibers using sheep embryos at each fetal week, and calf embryos at the latter two-thirds of intrauterine life. The result of his embryological study is summarized approximately as follows. Purkinje cells already appeared at the time when the whole myocardium was made up of spindle cells, where reorganization of protoplasm into fibrillary substance took place at the peripheral zone of the cells. From the beginning, Purkinje cells already demonstrated quite a different form from that of the spindle-shaped muscle cells. Schmaltz stated that the cells themselves had no cross-striations, and that already at this time cross-striated muscle fibrils developed between and over Purkinje cells. The number of Purkinje cells at the early embryonic stage was said to be no greater than in adult animals. During further developmental stages, the form of the cells became more distinct. According to him, an intricate intercellular cross-striated fibrillary net ran over poorly granulated cells, and then border cords appeared between the cells, and a fibrillary coat appeared over the cells. Marginal cross-striations, however, never entered the cells.

Schmaltz said that the fibrils did not belong to the cells but took their course from outside. They originally came from the spindle-shaped ordinary cardiac muscle cells and ran over and between the cells. From this reason, he named the fibrils running over and between the cells "intercellular fibrils," and the cords of the fibrils encircling the cells "border cords." He insisted that Purkinje cells, though having a fibrillary coat, were an independent and nonmuscular structure.

Schmaltz said nothing certain about the significance of Purkinje cells. He supposed, however, that the cells had something to do with a musculomotor final apparatus, and that Purkinje fibers subserved an important relationship with cardiac activity.

Toldt made a short remark on Purkinje fibers in his *Textbook of Histology* (3rd edition, 1888). He stated that Purkinje fibers were partly composed of slightly cross-striated contents, and were here and there replaced by a characteristic muscle substance. Frequently the cells appeared to be surrounded by a layer of cross-striated substance. The significance of the fibers was entirely unknown to him.

E. A. Schäfer wrote on Purkinje fibers in Quain's *Elements of Anatomy* (1893) as follows: the fibers were composed of muscle fibrils making a network by intervening with each other; the meshes of the net were filled with polygonal cells. In this way, muscle fibrils surrounded the cells and connected them together.

From Schäfer's view, the cells were peculiar muscle elements arrested in their development.

In A. Rauber's *Textbook of Human Anatomy* (1894), there is a short note on Purkinje fibers. He noticed that nets of gray fibers appeared under the endocardium in the human in the first month of life and also in many animals in the adult stage, and that the fibers were muscle cells, with embryonic characteristics standing side by side.

In the *Textbook of Histology* by Böhm and v. Davidoff, there is a short remark on Purkinje fibers. The authors stated that the fibers were composed of cells in which the protoplasm was transformed into cross-striated substance only at the periphery. The fibers were found in several animals but seldom in the human.

In 1897, in his textbook *Preciseness of Histology*, M. Duval argued strongly against the view of several authors that Purkinje fibers were composed of peculiar cells with muscle substance between the cells. He had the view, as did most other authors, that Purkinje fibers had no intervening substance but were exclusively made up of cells having cross-striated fibrils at the periphery. He claimed to have confirmed the transitions of Purkinje fibers to the ordinary cardiac muscle fibers.

Duval considered the cells as muscle fibers arrested in their development. He did not find the fibers in the human.

Romiti believed, as he described Purkinje fibers in his article "Treatise on Human Anatomy" (Vol. I, Part 4), that Purkinje cells were evidence that new cardiac cells were continuingly formed in the heart.

In 1898, R. Minervini[25] published his study "Particularity of Structure of the Cardiac Muscle Cells." He briefly referred to Purkinje fibers. He found the fibers mainly under the endocardium, but also in the myocardium. Purkinje cells were arranged in piles or in chains, and rarely appeared as isolated cells. The fibers continued directly to the ordinary cardiac muscle fibers. He did not find the fibers in the human.

Minervini was inclined to the view that Purkinje cells were altered muscle fibers belonging to the endocardium, or a special form of degenerated muscle cells not fully developed physiologically. The fibers were of a muscular nature, but a kind of hydropic muscle cells or incompletely developed and nonfunctioning cells.

In 1900, V. v. Ebner[26] commented briefly on Purkinje fibers in his study "Concerning Cement Lines of Cardiac Muscle Cells." He thought that the fibers were not typical cardiac muscle fibers at any developmental stage.

In 1901, under the title of "Continuity of Contractile Fibrils in Cardiac Muscle Cells," H. Hoyer[27] described Purkinje cells as having the following characteristics. Purkinje fibers were recognized in a special territory but had no apparent border. He considered the clear halo around a nucleus as an artificial product made by strong contraction of the nucleus as well as of the marginal portion of the cell body caused by reagents. The contractile fibrils not only existed in each cell, but bridged cell borders and continued further to the next cell. From the lengthwise fibrils arose lateral branches, which ran to the adjacent neighboring cells. Fibrils were composed of elements known in skeletal muscles. Purkinje fibers ran mostly in the subendocardium. From this superficial net of fibers, cords branched here and there and entered deeply the myocardium. The cells of the intramyocardial fibers gradually took on the characteristics of the ordinary muscle cells as they entered deeper, gradually losing their connecting tissue sheaths, and finally connected with the surrounding muscle cells.

Based on the above-mentioned findings, Hoyer gave the following significance to Purkinje fibers: Purkinje cells represented muscular elements in their developmental stage. Longitudinal growth of the cells was hindered, and hence the cells developed more in their width and thickness. As the heart grew, Purkinje cells gradually transformed into the ordinary cardiac muscle cells, particularly in the deeper layers of the myocardium.

At the Society of Biology, Marceau[28] made a brief communication on Purkinje fibers in which he described the embryonic development of the fibers in the sheep. He found the clearly differentiated Purkinje fibers already in a fetus of 10 cm. From the fact that the fibers already had a specific structure, he concluded that they were neither developmental arrests nor a transitional form to the ordinary cardiac muscle fibers, but a special form of cardiac muscle fibers having a hitherto unknown specific physiological function.

In the following year there appeared the study of H. K. Hofmann[29] entitled "Contribution to Knowledge on Purkinje Fibers in Cardiac Muscle." He found the fibers in the cow embryos, calf, cow, rabbit, rat, mouse, pigeon, chicken embryo and most clearly in the sheep, but he missed the fibers in the human embryo and in a 27-year-old adult human. In contrast to almost all the statements made before him, he argued that Purkinje fibers appeared not only in the endocardium and myocardium, but also frequently in the pericardium. Regarding the histology of the fibers, he emphasized that Purkinje fibers were, as A. v. Kölliker first indicated, composed of a series of muscle cells with cross-striated peripheral zones and beautiful nuclei, that the cells were not embedded in cross-striated intervening substance, and that fibrils continued from cell to cell. He again confirmed the fact that the fibers directly connected with the ordinary cardiac muscle fibers, and he described precisely these connections.

On the significance of the fibers, opposing the opinion that the fibers were the ordinary cardiac musculature arrested in the developmental process, he was inclined to consider that the cells were used for replacement of cardiac muscle fibers destroyed or unusable in the early stage. His findings on the transitions of the fibers to the ordinary cardiac muscle fibers, and on the active nuclear mitosis, seem to have led him to this opinion. He stressed, however, that further investigations must be made to demonstrate to what extent his opinion was correct.

The most recent work on Purkinje fibers I read was that of G. Moriya.[30] In 1904, in his study "Musculature of the Heart," he made a short remark on the fibers. He found the fibers only in the adult sheep, not seeing them in the sheep embryo, human, mammalian animals, birds, reptiles, amphibians and bone fishes he examined. According to him, Purkinje fibers were composed of many oval or elliptical cells, and sometimes formed a large group in the myocardium. The cells had a relatively large amount of protoplasm, and cross-striated fibrils running quite irregularly were embedded at the outer layer of the cells. In addition to the oval cells, there were cylindrical or relatively long cells which formed the ends of individual Purkinje fibers. They were difficult to differentiate histologically from the normal muscle fibers. Cement lines frequently appearing in the adult cardiac muscle fibers, but not in the embryonic fibers, were entirely absent in Purkinje fibers.

Moriya considered Purkinje fibers as the near-relative of embryonic muscle fibers on the basis of their similar characteristics of cell constitution, abundance of protoplasm and absence of cement lines.

In the recently published second edition of the *Textbook of Histology* by Stöhr (1905), there is the following description. In many mammalian animals (but seldom in the human, particularly in the sheep), there are Purkinje fibers composed of clear cells in series in the cardiac wall mostly under the endocardium. The peripheral layers of the cells contain cross-striated fibrils continuously running from cell to cell. The nuclei increase partly through mitosis and partly through amitosis (here cell division does not take place). The cells are regarded as a developing form to genuine cardiac muscle fibers, because they are gradually transformed into the genuine cardiac muscle fibers.

If the opinions of various authors concerning the physiological significance of Purkinje fibers, published until now, are briefly outlined in the order of the time periods, they are as follows:

(1) Purkinje (1845): A special motor apparatus with muscular walls.

(2) v. Kölliker (1852): An embryonic form; a peculiarly developed form of the cardiac muscle fibers in terms of the size of the cells.

(3) v. Heßling (1855): Purkinje corns are pieces of decomposed muscle cords or bundles in the ordinary cardiac muscle tissues.

(4) Reichert (1855): Netlike spread stretching muscle of the endocardium. The primitive muscle bundles behave somewhat differently from the ordinary cardiac musculature.

(5) Remak (1862): A special arrangement of muscle fibers in the firm and elastic endocardium for prevention of complete emptying of the ventricles.

(6) Aeby (1863): A form developing into all the cardiac muscle fibers.

(7) Eberth (1866): No comment on the significance.

(8) Obermeier (1867): A muscle apparatus designed to provide better endocardial tightening during ventricular contraction.

(9) Lehnert (1868): No significance other than that of the ordinary netlike arranged cardiac muscle fibers.

(10) Schweiggel-Seidel (1871): A special endocardial muscular layer equivalent to the entire vascular wall.

(11) Krause (1876): No comment on the significance of the fibers.

(12) Henle (1876): New layers participating in the formation of the muscular cardiac wall.

(13) Ranvier (1877): Embryonic muscle fibers arrested in their development.

(14) Gegenbauer (1877): Elements of cardiac muscle developed in a peculiar direction, but not remaining at their development.

(15) Schmaltz (1886): Not muscular cells; may be a musculomotor final apparatus, importantly related to cardiac activity.

(16) Schäfer (1893): Peculiar elements arrested in their development.

(17) Rauber (1894): Muscle cells with embryonic characteristics standing side by side.

(18) Duval (1897): Elements arrested in their development.

(19) Romiti: Germ for new cardiac muscle cells.

(20) Minervini (1898): Muscular elements, i.e. hydropic form of the ordinary cardiac muscle cells, or incompletely developed and non-functioning cells.

(21) Ebner (1900): Purkinje fibers are not typical cardiac muscle fibers at any developmental stage.

(22) Hoyer (1901): Muscle elements developmentally hindered in their longitudinal growth. They gradually become cardiac muscle cells as the heart grows up.

(23) Marceau (1901): Special system of cardiac muscle fibers of unknown function.

(24) Hofmann (1902): The cells are engaged in increment and regeneration of destroyed cardiac muscle fibers in the early stage.

(25) Moriya (1904): A near-relative of embryonic cardiac fibers.

(26) Stöhr (1905): Purkinje cells are regarded as a developing form to genuine cardiac muscle fibers.

Several other authors expressed no comments on the significance of Purkinje fibers.

As the above overview indicates, several hypotheses are repeatedly proposed. In consideration of my own findings, I will briefly criticize these hypotheses.

(I) One hypothesis insists that Purkinje fibers are especially related to the endocardium (Reichert, Remak, Obermeier, Schweiggel-Seidel). Remak's opinion (5) is in sharp contrast to the opinions of the other three authors.

He considered the fibers as a tool for reducing the contractility of the endocardium, whereas the other authors gave an opposite function to the fibers. Remak's view is based on his finding that the cardiac cavity of the animals with the fibers stayed open after death. His conclusion, however, is not valid, because the fibers are found in all the animals, including the human, independently of whether the ventricle stays open or not after death. Here, I will not discuss in detail why the suprapapillary space of the left ventricle does not contract completely. In the sense of Remak, it is quite obvious that incomplete contraction of the space has nothing to do with the physiological function of Purkinje fibers, because here only a few Purkinje fibers exist except for the main stem of the left bundle branch. As for the role of blood remaining for the closure of the atrioventricular valves, I just refer to Albrecht's[2] work.

Reichert (4) considered Purkinje fibers to be an endocardial tensor which tightened the endocardium at the time of ventricular contraction. He presumed this on the basis that Purkinje corns were arranged vertically to the endocardial surface. From my study, however, this assumption is invalid, because the arrangement of the corns and fibers are predominantly parallel to the endocardial surface.

Obermeier (8) agreed with Reichert's view and thought that Purkinje fibers might be related to endocardial function in terms of stretching or relaxation of the endocardium. He believed that he had found much-better-developed elastic endocardial layers in the animal hearts without Purkinje fibers than in the hearts with them. This argument is no longer true, because I already found Purkinje fibers in animals such as the human, cat and so on, in which Obermeier did not find the fibers, and hence there must be a stronger elastic fiber layer in the endocardium. Obermeier further considered the peculiar netlike arrangement of Purkinje fibers as an evidence for his hypothesis. This arrangement, however, does not exist in the same fashion in all the animals. In particular, the arrangement in the human left ventricle is entirely different from that in the sheep heart. This arrangement is explained in the other way and will be referred to later.

Schweiggel-Seidel's viewpoint is that the Purkinje system is a piece of equipment identical to the vascular musculature, namely to the muscular layer of the endocardium. His opinion, however, seems not acceptable to me, because Purkinje fibers take their course not only in the subendocardium but also frequently in the myocardium. Naturally, vascular musculature never leaves the vascular wall. Why should vascular musculature often run totally apart from the endocardium to which it belongs?

Anyway, I cannot agree with any of these hypotheses considering Purkinje fibers as an endocardial muscle, especially when not only histological findings or local arrangement but also the entire arrangement of the system is considered. If the fibers are to tighten or to stretch the endocardium, why are the muscles found only at the determined position? What purpose have the atrial segment, and the connecting bundle between the atrial and ventricular septums, which are not in the subendocardium?

(II) Eberth (7) and Lehnert (9) considered that Purkinje fibers had no other significance than representing the ordinary cardiac muscle fibers. I cannot accept this opinion, because the fibers exist with a definitely regular arrangement in all the mammalian animals examined, including the human. They are isolated from the ordinary myocardium by connective tissue, and are connected with the ordinary cardiac muscle fibers only at special sites. It is, therefore, inevitable to have an idea that a certain function must be ascribed to the system. The heart is a highly important organ which must perform regular pumping work restlessly and under every possible circumstance throughout life. Nature, which, as we already know from experience, made all the organs of the human and animals as purposefully as possible, must surely not neglect to do the best also for this vital organ. Now that nature has given to the heart of the mammalian animal and the human a special muscular system which more or less histologically differs from the myocardium, and which takes a course with a highly characteristic principle, this must have been done with a special intention. By the way, Eberth made his conclusion from an erroneous understanding of the histological structure of Purkinje fibers which is not surely true in the human. On the basis mentioned above, I am inclined to consider that the system has a characteristic physiological function. I will discuss this function later.

(III) Two authors regarded Purkinje fibers as a pathological phenomenon. v. Heßling (3), who first studied the fibers in detail, consequently came to the idea that Purkinje corns were pieces of decomposed muscle cords in the ordinary cardiac muscle tissue. Minervini (20) considered the fibers to be either a hydropic form of the ordinary cardiac muscle fibers, or incompletely developed cells with no physiological function. This opinion is rejected, because, in order to label a tissue as pathological, an uncommon finding must be made. Constant tissues, such as Purkinje fibers, appearing as a definite system in all the hearts during the whole life without exception, cannot be called pathological. Also, a tissue showing no degenerative signs cannot be identified as functionless.

(IV) Schmaltz (15) gave Purkinje cells a special significance. Regarding the cells — not Purkinje fibers — as a piece of musculomotor equipment, he speculated that Purkinje cells played an important role in cardiac activity. This speculation was based on his own histological understanding that Purkinje fibers were composed not only of muscular tissue, but of characteristic, nonmuscular and large transparent cells and of special intercellular fibrillary bundles encircling the cells. Because this understanding was disproved by many authors, including myself, and because the fiber system existed in the same arrangement in all animals examined and also in the human being, although Purkinje "corns" or "cells" existed in certain mammalian animals and the human not in the form characteristic of the ungulates, no special significance apart from the fiber system could be given to the "corns" or "cells."

(V) Many authors, such as v. Kölliker, Gegenbauer, Ranvier, Schäfer, Rauber, Duval and Moriya, commented only on the histological characteristics of Purkinje fibers or cells, offering nothing of physiological significance. All the authors explained Purkinje fibers in connection with embryonic cardiac muscle cells. Whether they gave Purkinje fibers the same physiological significance as the ordinary cardiac muscle fibers or not, I cannot say anything certain from their statements. When Ranvier (13), Schäfer (16) and Duval (18) said that Purkinje fibers were embryonic muscle fibers arrested in their development, they supposedly considered that the fibers had peculiar structures either of cardiac muscle fibers later capable of becoming normal cardiac muscle fibers, or of functionally inefficient elements. From my viewpoint mentioned above, both are not true. Marceau already correctly emphasized that a muscle fiber system which had its special structure from the early embryonic period throughout life must have a special function.

v. Kölliker (2) and Gegenbauer (14) understood Purkinje cells somewhat differently, regarding the cells to be a peculiarly developed form of the cardiac muscle fibers. They expressed nothing, however, about the function.

(VI) Many authors considered Purkinje fibers as a developmental form of cardiac muscle fibers.

Aeby (6) was the first to offer this opinion. He believed that all the cardiac muscle fibers developed from Purkinje cells. In addition to the well-known connection of Purkinje fibers with the cardiac muscle fibers, he regarded the "jointed" muscle fibers, which he claimed to find in animals and humans at all their ages, as evidence for his opinion.

Henle (12) considered Purkinje fibers as new layers related to the construction of the muscular portion of the cardiac wall. His idea is mainly based on his finding of the transitions of Purkinje fibers into the cardiac muscle fibers.

Romiti (19) and Hoyer (22) had more or less the same view as Henle, which was quoted in Stöhr's *Textbook of Histology*.

Hofmann (24) considered that Purkinje fibers were probably destined to construct the cardiac muscle fibers. According to him, Purkinje fibers must concern either growth of the cardiac muscle or replacement of the cardiac muscle fibers which would soon die or become useless. He reached this view mainly from the transitions he pictured between Purkinje fibers and the cardiac muscle fibers as well as from numerous nuclear mitoses he found in Purkinje cells.

As seen here, almost all the recent publications have held this view, which is regarded as the most prevalent at the present time.

To me, it is not necessary to emphasize that this view is no longer acceptable. The transition pictures, which played an important role for many authors, do not indicate at all a transformation of Purkinje fibers into the cardiac muscle fibers.

Aeby considered that all the cardiac muscle fibers originated from Purkinje cells. From his viewpoint, Purkinje fibers decreased in number as the cardiac muscle fibers increased, and finally they disappeared. This is not true at all. Purkinje fibers continue to exist as a system which is found in all the heart of mammalian animals throughout life, and the extent of the system does not seem to change at all with ageing. Through his exact study of the sheep and calf embryos of various fetal stages, Schmaltz demonstrated that the amount of Purkinje cells was not greater at any stage of fetal life than in the adult heart. I also studied the system in human embryos of various ages and, in an approximately three-month-old fetus, observed the system existing already with a typically completed course. For this reason, I cannot agree with Aeby's viewpoint.

However far the other authors, Henle, Romiti, Hoyer, Hofmann and Stöhr, might go in their understanding, I cannot agree with them. Authors such as Aeby regarded Purkinje cells as constructing cells of all the cardiac muscle fibers. If this is so, it must be admitted that the ordinary cardiac muscle fibers are products of two completely different constructing cells, namely ordinary myoblasts and Purkinje cells. This is quite difficult to understand. At any rate, the hypothesis regarding Purkinje cells as a developing form to the cardiac muscle fibers seems to me not sufficiently grounded. All the investigators until now have failed to find Purkinje fibers in the atria. In order to evaluate the physiological significance of Purkinje fibers without prejudice, this striking fact should be taken into consideration, because the atrium, as well as the ventricle, requires constructing cells for its muscle fibers.

Much more important to me is that, from my study, Purkinje fibers exist only at regular and similar sites in all the examined animals, and are separated by a connective tissue sheath throughout most of the course from the ordinary cardiac muscle fibers. Formation of younger cardiac muscle fibers to replace extinct elements, therefore, could take place only where a connective tissue sheath does not exist, and where Purkinje fibers are connected to the ordinary cardiac muscle fibers. None of the investigators, however, has ever recognized the appearance of younger muscle fibers at such a site. Only Hofmann insisted that he saw the young muscle fibers originating from Purkinje cells and reported: "When cardiac muscle cells are unbiasedly observed, an idea comes that there are two different kinds of cardiac muscle fibers, namely those looking dark, more striated with small nuclei and those looking clearer with large nuclei. I think the latter are related to Purkinje fibers" (p. 500). He wrote in the summary of his result: "The cardiac muscle fibers develop from Purkinje cells and the cardiac muscle bundles from Purkinje fibers, which distinguish themselves by a large form, a clearer color and larger nuclei for a longer time." I did not confirm this finding. As I already mentioned in my anatomical chapter, I also noticed clear spots in the calf hearts. Through my exact study, the spots mostly appeared at the transitional sites from Purkinje fibers to the ordinary cardiac muscle fibers. Appearance of nuclear division, at least of amitosis, does not demonstrate productive or degenerative activity of Purkinje cells, because duplicated nuclei are frequently found in the sarcoplasm of the ordinary cardiac muscle fibers.

Finally, it is strange if regeneration takes place at the mostly exposed layer where regeneration is easily damaged by endocardial infection.

Consequently, I conclude that all the advocated viewpoints on the physiological significance of Purkinje fibers are invalid. Only the statement of v. Kölliker and others that Purkinje fibers are characteristically developed cardiac muscle fibers is not yet refuted. Until now, however, nothing sure has been mentioned about the function.

II. Author's Hypothesis Concerning the Physiological Function of the Atrioventricular Connecting System

Based on my topographic–anatomical and histological findings, I now believe that I can give a clear explanation of the heretofore unknown function of Purkinje fibers. My explanation comes from the fact that Purkinje fibers are nothing other than the terminal ramifications of the muscular connecting system, of which only the part between the atrium and the ventricle has been known up to now. Therefore, the function of Purkinje fibers must be the same as that of the atrioventricular bundle.

Whenever any hypothesis is proposed, the system involved should be taken into consideration as a whole. Moreover, a conclusion derived from the anatomical architecture must eventually accord with the results of physiological experiments regarding the system.

The first question is whether the connecting system containing the terminal ramifications exists in all the hearts of human beings, mammals and birds. The existence of the main bundle of the connecting system, i.e. the atrioventricular bundle, has been confirmed in rats, mice, rabbits, cats, dogs, lions, monkeys and human beings (except for the hearts of cold-blooded animals) through the studies of Stanley Kent, W. His Jr., R. Retzer, K. Braeunig and M. Humblet. Likewise, the terminal ramifications, i.e. Purkinje fibers, have already been found in the hearts of sheep, calves, cows, pigs, horses, goats, deer, dogs, cats, rabbits, hedgehogs and Mustela foina, and in the hearts of birds such as pigeons, fowls and geese. The existence of genuine Purkinje fibers in nonungulate animals has been questioned by many authors, and their existence in the human heart has been denied by almost all the authors. My recent investigations, however, have indicated that such a view is not accurate, and have demonstrated that a similar well-developed connecting system can be found in the hearts of human beings, dogs, cats, rabbits, guinea pigs, sheep, calves, cows and pigeons. The histological peculiarities of the terminal ramifications, i.e. Purkinje fibers, are not as conspicuous in human beings, dogs, cats, rabbits and so forth as in the ungulates. Because I have found that the connecting system in many different animals always takes a similar course, I am now fully convinced that the connecting system exists in all species of mammals and birds. I emphasized previously that it is not always easy to identify this system, particularly in smaller mammals and birds, because these muscle fibers are very small, and because histological differentiation between the terminal ramifications of the connecting system and the ordinary ventricular musculature is almost impossible. This was the case in the rat heart.

Except for slight histological differences and variations in the peripheral terminal ramifications of the system, there is surprising regularity in the architecture of the atrioventricular connecting bundle in all the animals examined. Using the sheep heart as an example, I will again briefly summarize the regularity of the connecting system.

The atrioventricular connecting system forms a relatively large, complicated network of muscular tissues immediately above the atrioventricular fibrocartilaginous septum. We call this complicated network the "node" (Knoten). From this node, short bundles of muscle fibers, arranged more or less parallel to each other, posteriorly extend approximately to the front end of the coronary sinus, where they connect with the ordinary atrial muscle fibers. On the other side, the node becomes much thinner, advances anteriorly, and continues to the ventricular segment of the connecting bundle. After penetrating the fibrocartilaginous septum, the bundle enters the ventricular septum. The histological difference between the muscle fibers of the connecting bundle and the atrial and ventricular muscle fibers is not mentioned here. After the bundle enters the ventricular septum, it divides into two bundle branches. The left bundle branch quickly reaches the left endocardium and takes a course downward as a closed bundle surrounded by a connective tissue sheath. The left bundle branch first divides into many bundles at a level considerably lower than where it begins. The largest bundle enters tendinous fiber-like cords, passes through the ventricular cavity, and extends to the anterior and posterior papillary muscles. From the papillary muscles, the muscle bundles spread in every direction in the subendocardium just like the roots of a tree. Subendocardial twigs from the papillary muscles partly spread along the ventricular wall and extend to the ventricular base as well as to the apex. The remaining bundles of the left bundle branch not entering the cords extend in a similar manner. The finest terminal ramifications are connected with the ordinary ventricular musculature in the subendocardium or in the myocardium.

The right bundle branch gradually approaches the right ventricular subendocardium, but usually does not reach the endocardium. It is entirely surrounded by connective tissue and proceeds downward about 2 cm within the myocardium, where it reaches a relatively large muscular trabeculation. The trabeculation leads the bundle branch to the anterior papillary muscle or to the adjacent parietal wall. Here, the right bundle branch suddenly spreads in many directions, toward the cardiac base as well as the cardiac apex, and spreads beneath the endocardium. The numerous finest terminal ramifications connect directly with the ordinary ventricular muscle fibers, particularly in the subendocardium.

Along the long course from the atrial bundle to the finest terminal ramifications in the ventricular wall, the connecting bundle, surrounded by connective tissues, is totally isolated from the myocardium and at no place does it connect with the ordinary ventricular musculature. *The connecting bundle is a closed system like a tree. This tree is rooted in the atrial septum, the stem and the main branches penetrate the fibrocartilaginous septum and the ventricular septum, their peripheral branches reach the parietal wall and the papillary muscles through the false tendinous fibers, and finally the thinnest twigs spread as the terminal ramifications of the connecting bundle.*

This architecture completely corresponds to that of the other ductal or parenchymal systems with roots and branches, such as the respiratory, circulatory and nervous systems in animals. In all these systems, gases or fluids are transported or impulse conduction takes place. *From the structural viewpoint, the connecting system also represents a transporting or conducting pathway. Because the pathway is not a ductal, but a continuously related protoplasmic cord, conduction of excitation impulses surely must take place there.*

I will not refer in detail to the theories regarding the neurogenic or myogenic origin of the rhythmical activity of the heart. I will refer only to Engelmann's[31] precise and concise treatise ("Myogenic Theory and Innervation of the Heart"). He is an enthusiastic supporter of the myogenic theory, which is gaining ground against the neurogenic theory. The myogenic theory takes the view that, in all animals, rhythmical cardiac activity is inherent in the heart muscle cells, in the embryo as well as in the adult, that cardiac activity is independent of the extracardiac as well as the intracardiac nervous system, and that the nervous system plays only a secondary role in cardiac regulation. The myogenic theory insists further that the cardiac impulse is conducted not through nerve fibers but through the block of muscle fibers* that extend between the atrium and the ventricle.

With regard to impulse conduction, my anatomical observations of the connecting system absolutely agree with the results of physiological experiments performed by the supporters of the myogenic theory.

In impulse conduction, the interval between the atrial systole (As) and the ventricular systole (Vs) is important, because without this interval (As–Vs) the heart cannot maintain its normal function continuously. The As–Vs interval is as long as the duration of atrial systole, so that the next ventricular systole begins just after the termination of the previous atrial systole. Because the velocity of impulse conduction through nerves is very fast, it is not possible that impulses from the atrium to the ventricle are conducted through a neural pathway.

The supporters of the myogenic theory have based their explanation of this relatively slow impulse conduction (As–Vs interval) on the hypothesis that the muscle fibers of the connecting bundle are similar to embryonic muscle fibers, which conduct the impulse slower than the ordinary cardiac muscle fibers. Engelmann,[31] for example, in his above-mentioned treatise (p. 231) said: "As already stated above, the block of muscle fibers is histologically markedly different from the ventricular and atrial muscle fibers, and is relatively similar to the architecture of smooth muscles

---

*Blockfasern

and embryonic cardiac muscles. As G. Fano[32] demonstrated by direct measurement of the embryonic cardiac muscle of warm-blooded animals, the velocity of motor conduction is much slower than that in the ventricular and the atrial walls of the adult heart. For example, the velocity was 6–11.5 Mm in a chicken of three days of age at 39°C, whereas, in a developed heart, it was 50 Mm or more in a frog, and would be much faster in warm-blooded animals. It is a logical consequence, therefore, particularly because no counterevidence has been found, that the block of muscle fibers has a slower conduction velocity. As far as conductivity is concerned, the block of muscle fibers stays at the embryonic stage."

Although this interpretation seems to be reasonable at first glance, I do not agree with it. Contrary to the view of the physiologists, I believe that conduction velocity is much more rapid in the muscle fibers of the connecting bundle. My opinion is based upon the characteristic course of the atrioventricular connecting bundle. It has generally been believed that the atrioventricular bundle connects directly with the ventricular musculature soon after penetrating the thin atrioventricular fibrous septum. In reality, however, the bundle reaches the papillary muscles and the parietal walls via a long course. It must be stressed that an impulse wave must travel a considerably long distance from the atrial musculature before it arrives at the ventricular musculature. For example, I estimate the distance of the connecting bundle of a sheep heart at about 4–6 cm or much longer. *In my opinion, this characteristic architecture, by which the impulse wave is transported directly to the remotest segments of the ventricular walls through the closed pathways, serves to convey the excitation impulse as simultaneously as possible to all sites of the ventricular walls.* For this reason, the velocity of an impulse wave in the connecting bundle must be faster than in the ordinary ventricular muscles. If the velocity is slower, the characteristic architecture of the connecting system, including the terminal ramifications, would be entirely useless, and only a single connection of the atrioventricular bundle between the atrium and the ventricle would be sufficient to transmit an impulse. Because the connecting bundle was erroneously thought to be short, and the muscle fibers of the connecting bundle were thought to be connected with the ordinary ventricular muscle fibers immediately after entering the ventricular septum, the physiologists were forced to accept an idea of slower impulse conduction velocity in the connecting bundle and to explain this as a consequence of the embryonic characteristics of these muscle fibers. This idea, however, is not valid, because the embryonic cardiac muscle fibers never show the form typical of Purkinje cells. From the beginning, Purkinje cells develop as they do. A scarcity of myofibrils and an abundance of protoplasm are the only similarities in these two types of fibers.

It should be emphasized, moreover, that each segment of the connecting system is histologically varied and that, therefore, the functional ability of each segment will differ somewhat. Further experimental-physiological studies will clarify what significance each segment has in conducting excitation. I merely express the opinion that the connecting bundle serves to transport impulses from the atrium to the ventricle in a normal heart, and that impulses are transmitted not slowly but rapidly in this system at least in the ventricular bundles. I must admit the possibility, however, that inhibition of impulse conduction takes place in the "node."

Under pathological conditions, the functional ability of the connecting bundle as a whole or of each of its segments is likely to change, as demonstrated by many recent physiological experiments, especially Hering's careful studies.

Embryological observations have also been significant. In the works of His,[8] for example, the following description (p. 18) is found: "On the fourth or fifth day after hatching, a transformation which determines the ultimate partitioning of the heart occurs ... . Between the fourth and fifth days, the ventricular muscular wall begins to change. The hitherto vesicular cells take a fibrillary structure and then the reticular arrangement of muscular trabeculations appears in the inner wall of the ventricle.

From this moment, the characteristics of cardiac contraction change. Formerly, contraction took the form of a peristaltic wave with uniform velocity over the cardiac tube. Now, however, contraction begins at the caval veins, and after a small delay it moves over the atrium. Then, again, after a pause, the ventricles start to contract simultaneously, and contraction spreads to the aortic bulbus in a peristaltic movement ... . Except for the special movement of the bulbus, which loses its musculature in mammals, and the movement of the sinus, which is included in the atrium, the form of contraction of the chicken embryo is similar to that of the adult bird and mammal."

Hering[33] quoted this observation and remarked: "A special arrangement in the atrioventricular bundle connecting the atrium and the ventricle possibly regulates the conduction delay." His's statement is very interesting to me, because it made me speculate that, at the very moment the atrioventricular bundle develops in the chicken heart, the chicken heart shows such a particular arrangement like a mammalian heart and changes the peristaltic contraction into the typical ventricular contraction. From His's statement, I assume that, just at this moment, on the ventricular inner wall there appear the muscular trabeculations in the reticular arrangement characteristic of the terminal ramifications of the connecting system. Future embryological studies of the development of the connecting system will indicate whether my assumption is valid. In spite of great time-consuming efforts, using many human embryos kindly given to me by Professor Gasser, I have not been able to solve this problem.

Before ending this chapter, I must make mention of the *nerve bundles*. As I particularly emphasized in the anatomical chapter, the atrioventricular connecting bundle in the calf heart is accompanied by a highly recognizable nerve bundle closely entangled with the muscle bundle, and even containing ganglion cells in the ventricular septum. I could also confirm several small nerve bundles in the sheep heart, but could not find any nerve bundles worth mentioning in the hearts of human beings, dogs, cats and so on. It cannot be denied, however, that the connecting system in the hearts of these animals is accompanied by very fine nerve bundles. The nerve bundles accompanying the connecting system have not been known before.

Now a question arises: What is the physiological function of these nerve bundles? Here, I merely mention that the physiologists consider that rhythmical cardiac activity does not depend upon the intra- or the extracardiac nervous system, but that cardiac activity is automatically generated by excitation of the cardiac muscle cells; in other words, the nervous system only functions to regulate cardiac activity in order to adapt to various external and internal life conditions.

With my anatomical observations alone, I cannot comment on the question raised by Engelmann in his treatise cited above. I must be satisfied with confirming the facts.

D. Summary of the Results

The essential findings of my study are as follows:

(1) In the hearts of human beings and all other mammals and birds (dog, cat, rabbit, guinea pig, sheep, calf, cattle and pigeon), Purkinje fibers or their equivalents exist. The histological characteristics are described precisely.

(2) In the human heart and in those of all the other animals examined, Purkinje fibers and their equivalents form the terminal ramifications of the muscle fiber system connecting the atrial and the ventricular musculature; this connection was already partly described by His as the atrioventricular bundle.

(3) The connecting system containing the terminal ramifications is arranged systematically in the hearts of humans and of all the other animals investigated. In spite of small differences, the arrangement is generally identical among all the animals. The topographic course of this system is described precisely for each animal species.

(4) In human beings, and in all the other animals examined, the connecting system originates in the atrial septum, penetrates the atrioventricular fibrous septum, and finally reaches various portions of the ventricular wall as the terminal ramifications. The connecting system is always separated from the ordinary cardiac musculature by connective tissues. The system is a closed muscle bundle that resembles a tree, having a beginning, or root, and branches. At no place does the muscle bundle of the connecting system connect with the ordinary cardiac musculature

during the bundle's course to the terminal ramifications. The system connects with the ordinary ventricular musculature for the first time at the terminal ramifications.

(5) The connecting system is already well developed at a relatively early human embryonic stage, and it remains unchanged lifelong, except for growth in size.

(6) When the heart is affected by hypertrophic or atrophic processes, the connecting system seems not to be proportionally influenced as is the ordinary myocardium.

(7) All the topographical, histological and biological peculiarities of this muscular system indicate that the system does not participate in the pumping activity of the ordinary cardiac muscle. In agreement with the view advocated by Gaskell, Engelmann and others, and supported by Hering's elaborate experiments, the peculiarities of the connecting system indicate that excitation is conducted by this system and that the system controls the coordinated movement of the cardiac chambers. The prolongation of excitation conduction in the connecting system as compared with that of the ordinary cardiac musculature, a fact apparent to the physiologists, is fully explained not only by the special histological structures of the muscle fibers of this system, but also by the characteristic topology of the connecting bundle and its twigs.

E. Instructions Regarding the Method of Cutting the Atrioventricular Bundle in Animal Experiments

Attempts had already been made by many physiologists to cut or to interrupt the atrioventricular bundle to examine its physiological significance in a living and beating heart that had been artificially perfused. As there have been no reliable clues — except for the clue proposed by Hering — for conducting successful experiments, it seems to me that I should refer to this point in detail.

Because most of the experiments have been conducted using dogs, I utilized a dog heart. The following statements, nonetheless, are also applicable to other animal hearts, as this portion of the connecting bundle is located uniformly in each animal species.

In order to cut successfully the connecting bundle, it is mandatory to choose a site where the bundle can easily be accessed and where the bundle has not yet divided into the bundle branches. Hering chose the site beneath the membranous septum and, through experiments, proved the correctness of his choice. We also confirmed the correctness of his choice of site by examining the experimental objects microscopically.

Because the bundle already begins to branch to the left and to the right beneath the membranous septum, it is absolutely necessary to select a site containing the atrioventricular bundle before it branches. How can one identify the site correctly?

The membranous septum can clearly be seen by transilluminating the ventricular septum in the human and dog hearts. The membranous septum, however, is not sufficiently reliable as a key for use in an experimental operation, because it is not always recognizable in an experiment.

Based on my own observations, I recommend the following procedure. As shown in Fig. *A*, the annuli of the septal and the anterior leaflet of the tricuspid valve meet at the center of the membranous septum. This point (Fig. *A*, *a*) and the annulus of the septal tricuspid valvar leaflet (*ab*), as well as an imaginary vertical line downward from the point *a* (*ac*), are very important. Between the line (*ab*)–(*ac*) lies the beginning of the ventricular segment of the connecting bundle, running as a closed bundle. Interruption of this particular site offers a definite guarantee for a successful experiment.

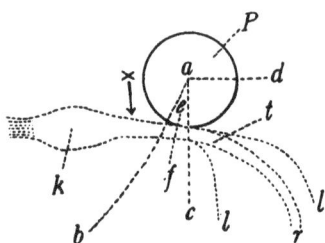   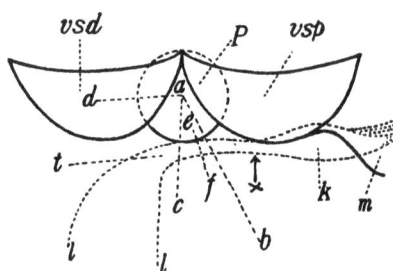

Fig. *A*   Fig. *B*

P = the membranous septum; *a* = approximately the center of the membranous septum, where the annuli of the septal (*ab*) and the anterior (*ad*) leaflet of the tricuspid valve meet; *ac* = an imaginary vertical line downward from the point *a*; *ef* = the line of incision; *k* = Knoten, or node, i.e. the atrial segment of the connecting bundle; *x* = approximately the boundary between the atrium and the ventricle; *t* = the site of bifurcation of the bundle into the wider left (*ll*) and the narrower right (*r*) bundle branch; *vsd* and *vsp* = the right coronary and the noncoronary aortic leaflet respectively; *m* = the anterior mitral leaflet.

The best way to achieve interruption of the bundle is via a parietal incision in the right atrial wall. An opening incision of the right atrium is made behind the right atrial appendage, or the orifice of the superior caval vein to the right atrium is better extended anteroinferiorly. From this incision, one can recognize point *a*, where the septal and the anterior tricuspid leaflet meet, even in a living heart. At point *e* (Fig. *A*), which is located between the septal tricuspid valvar annulus (*ab*) and the imaginary vertical line (*ac*) and approximately 2 mm below point *a*, a stab incision is made (using a sharp knife). The incision is then extended downward 5 mm along the line (*ab*), or better yet, along the line (*ef*). As shown in Fig. *A*, the line (*ef*) runs midway between the lines (*ab*) and (*ac*), dividing the angle (*bac*) into two equal parts. The knife must reach the left ventricular side. Care should be taken not to injure the left ventricular free wall by stabbing too deeply. Fig. *B* shows the incision line as seen from the left ventricular side.

It must be emphasized that, if the results are to be utilized in physiological experiments, the incision should carefully be checked microscopically. Depending on the individual variation in the extension of the membranous septum, the connecting bundle is only partly, or not at all, interrupted in some cases. It is recommended in microscopical examinations that about 12-μ-thick serial horizontal sections of the incised portion be made, and that every seventh or eighth section be regularly mounted and stained using the van Gieson method.

Finally, in finishing this work, I extend my sincere appreciation to my respected teacher, Professor L. Aschoff, for his valuable suggestions and for the very generous support he extended to me in performing this study.

Marburg a. L., 24 December 1905

Plates

Topography of the atrioventricular system of the human and mammalian hearts

In the following plates, I–V, photographs of the hearts are shown. On the tracing paper, the course of the connecting bundle is drawn red together with its bundle branches, twigs and terminal ramifications. As the course of the connecting bundle varies considerably in each animal, even in the same species, one or two arbitrarily selected examples for animals and humans are shown. Detailed descriptions are given in the text. As examples of individual differences of the course of the left bundle branch, two left ventricles of the human hearts (Figs. 1 & 2, Plate I) as well as two left ventricles of the bovine hearts (Figs. 1 & 2, Plate V) are illustrated.

Plate I

Fig. 1. The left ventricle of the human heart

The left ventricle is opened in its anterior wall between the two papillary muscles from the aortic orifice to the apex, and the opening is widened to both sides.

a = aorta
p = pulmonary artery
acd = right coronary artery
vsd = right coronary leaflet of the aortic valve
vsp = noncoronary leaflet of the aortic valve

mpa = anterior papillary muscle

mpp = posterior papillary muscle

vma = anterior leaflet of the mitral valve

vmp = posterior leaflet of the mitral valve

    k = Knoten, i.e. the node, the atrial segment of the atrioventricular connecting bundle

    x = dividing site of the connecting bundle into the left and right bundle branches

   + = terminal ramifications of the connecting bundle

  ++ = a 2-cm-long tendinous fiber-like cord of horsehair thickness, running upward from the tip of the posterior papillary muscle through the ventricular cavity and attaching to the upper posterior portion of the ventricular septum. This cord leads a small twig of the left bundle branch from the papillary muscle to the wall portion mentioned above.

Fig. 2. The left ventricle of the human heart

a, p, acd, vsd, vsp, vma, vmp, k, x, + and *mpp* have the same meanings as in Fig. 1, Plate I.

   as = left atrial appendage

  ats = left atrium

mpa′ = bigger half of the lengthwise-sectioned anterior papillary muscle which is retracted up toward the atrial chamber

 mpa = smaller half of the anterior papillary muscle which stays at its natural position

  ++ = a retrogradely running subendocardial terminal ramification of the connecting bundle

  xx = apical portion of the ventricular septum is cut away here.

Plate II

Fig. 1. The right ventricle of the human heart

A part (*pw*) of the parietal wall is strongly lifted upward and another part of the parietal wall is retracted posteriorly. A part of the opened left ventricle (*lk*) is visible.

    mpm = medial papillary muscle

    mpa = anterior papillary muscle

    mpp = posterior papillary muscle

    vtm = septal leaflet of the tricuspid valve, most of which is resected

    vta = anterior leaflet of the tricuspid valve

    vtl = posterior leaflet of the tricuspid valve

    atd = right atrium

    sw = ventricular septum

    c = supraventricular crest

    k = Knoten, i.e. the node of the connecting bundle

    rs = right bundle branch of the connecting bundle

    ++ = a retrogradely running twig of the right bundle branch

Fig. 2. The left ventricle of the dog heart

This heart is opened in the same fashion as that in Fig. 1, Plate I. Two groups of tendinous fiber-like cords (*sa* and *sp*) are seen in the left ventricle. The cords, connecting each other and forming a net, attach to the anterior and posterior papillary muscles. Not only these cords but also other isolated cords (*s*) carry muscle fibers of the ventricular bundle of the connecting system.

a, *acd*, *vsd*, *vsp*, *mpa*, *mpp*, *vma*, *vmp*, *as*, *ats*, *x*, + and *k* are the same as in Fig. 1 or Fig. 2, Plate I.

    vss = left coronary leaflet of the aortic valve

    sf = tendinous fibers for the mitral valve

    ++ = retrogradely running terminal ramifications of the left bundle branch

    x = vertical line

Plate III

Fig. 1. The right ventricle of the dog heart

Almost the whole parietal wall is separated from the septum and lifted upward. *atd*, *vtm*, *vta*, *vtl*, *mpm*, *mpp*, *pw* and *sw* are the same as in Fig. 1, Plate II.

sc = coronary sinus

p = pulmonary orifice

xx = attachment line of the septal leaflet of the tricuspid valve, a part of which is cut away

k = Knoten, i.e. the node of the connecting bundle

rs = right bundle branch of the connecting system

s = a big twig of the right bundle branch enters tendinous fiber-like cord (*s*) which shortly divides into two twigs (*s'*) and attaches to the parietal wall. From this attachment, the terminal ramifications of the connecting system spread in all directions. This small cord (s) can be seen in almost all the dog hearts, although its course varies. In several hearts, it divides into numerous twigs, which, connecting each other and forming several net meshes in the ventricular cavity, attach to different sites of the parietal wall and, from these sites, spread as the subendocardial terminal ramifications.

+ = terminal ramification

++ = a retrogradely running twig of the right bundle branch

The following comment should be noted here: as mentioned in the text, I could not use any fresh hearts for macroscopical description of the connecting bundle of dogs. Later, however, I had several opportunities to examine the fresh dog hearts. The subendocardial terminal ramifications of the connecting system are seen relatively well in most cases and even very clearly in several cases, as in the ungulate hearts. Also in the dog heart, they mostly consist of narrow and long fibers, but partly of wide membranes, which connect or divide each other, forming nets. Net meshes, however, are usually not as tight as in the sheep heart. These terminal ramifications are recognized everywhere in the subendocardium of both the ventricles.

Fig. 2. The left ventricle of the sheep heart

a, *p*, *acd*, *vsp*, *vsd*, *vma*, *vmp*, *mpa*, *mpp*, *as*, *ats* and ++ are the same as in Figs. 1 and 2, Plate I.

rk = right ventricle

sf = tendinous fibers attaching to the anterior papillary muscle

n = clearly visible subendocardial net formation of the terminal ramifications of the connecting bundle, i.e. Purkinje fibers

ls = left bundle branch of the connecting system

s = a relatively big tendinous fiber-like cord exists in almost all the sheep hearts. The left bundle branch of the connecting bundle enters this cord. The left bundle branch goes through the cord and then through its twigs to both the papillary muscles and to their adjacent wall portions.

Plate IV

Fig. 1. The right ventricle of the sheep heart

This heart was processed in the same fashion as the right ventricle of the dog heart (Fig. 1, Plate III).

atd, vta, vtm, vtl, mpa, mpm, mpp, sc, k, rs, p and *sw* are the same as for the right ventricle of the dog heart.

s = a constantly existing muscle trabeculation of the sheep heart, which stretches from the septum (*sw*) to the parietal wall (*pw*). In this figure, the trabeculation is cut in its middle. The trabeculation (*s'*) at the parietal wall is the continuation of the trabeculation (*s*). The right bundle branch always enters this muscle trabeculation. At the anterior papillary muscle or its vicinity, to which the trabeculation attaches, the right bundle branch is, for the first time, divided into numerous terminal ramifications, which run in all directions and spread not only to the parietal wall but also retrogradely to all the septal surfaces to form nets everywhere.

n = highly visible net formation of Purkinje fibers which is schematically reproduced on the tracing paper.

Fig. 2. The right ventricle of the bovine heart

Most of the parietal wall is separated from the septum and opened to the side. The remainder of the parietal wall is retracted posteriorly.

atd, vta, vtl, mpa, mpm, mpp, sc, sw, k and *rs* are the same as in Fig. 1, Plate IV.

> *vtm* = septal leaflet of the tricuspid valve; large portion of the leaflet is cut away at its base.
>
> + = a terminal ramification of the right bundle branch
>
> ++ = a retrogradely running twig of the right bundle branch, which goes back to the septum through the constantly existing muscle trabeculation (*s*) of the bovine heart and spreads in the septum.
>
> *s'* = small trabeculations extending between the parietal wall and the septum, which carry Purkinje fibers

a', *b'*, *c'*, *d'* and so on are continuations of the subendocardial terminal ramifications *a*, *b*, *c*, *d* and so on.

Subendocardial net formations are actually much tighter and complicated than illustrated on the tracing paper.

Plate V

Fig. 1. The left ventricle of the bovine heart

a, *acd*, *vsp*, *vsd*, *vma*, *vmp*, *mpa*, *mpp*, *sf*, *ats* and *ls* are the same as in Fig. 2, Plate III. *sa* and *sp* are tendinous fiber-like cords leading main twigs of the left bundle branch to the anterior and posterior papillary muscles.

> ++ = a terminal ramification of the left bundle branch running retrogradely toward the base of the left ventricle

Fig. 2. The left ventricle of the bovine heart

a, *acd*, *vsp*, *vsd*, *vma*, *vmp*, *mpa*, *mpp*, *sf*, *ats*, *sa*, *sp*, ++ and *ls* are the same as in Fig. 1, Plate V.

> *as* = left atrial appendage
>
> *rk* = right ventricle
>
> *sf'* = tendinous fibers for both leaflets of the mitral valve
>
> *s* = a short tendinous fiber-like cord bridging an intertrabecular gap and conveying a Purkinje fiber
>
> *p* = pulmonary orifice

Plate I

Fig 1.

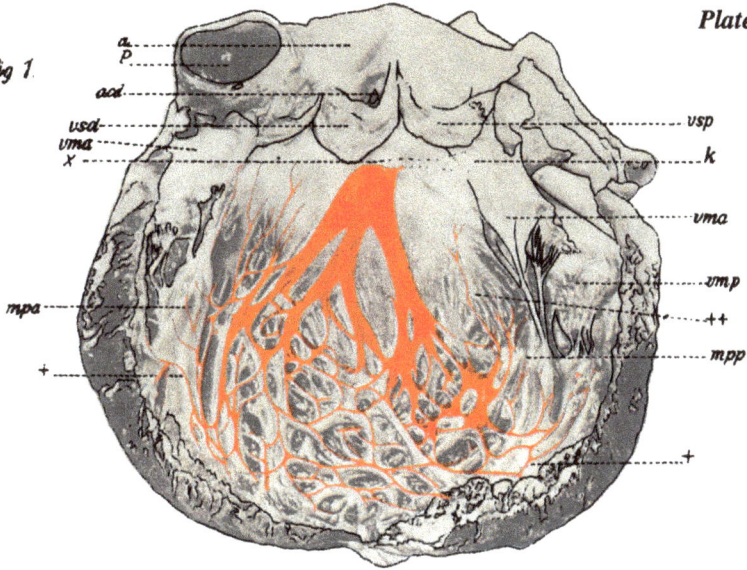

Fig 2.

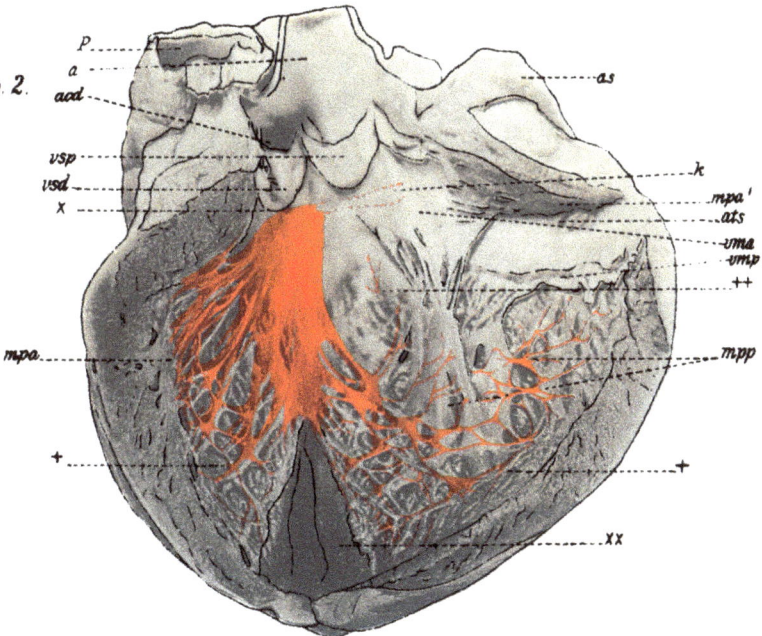

Plate II

Fig. 1.

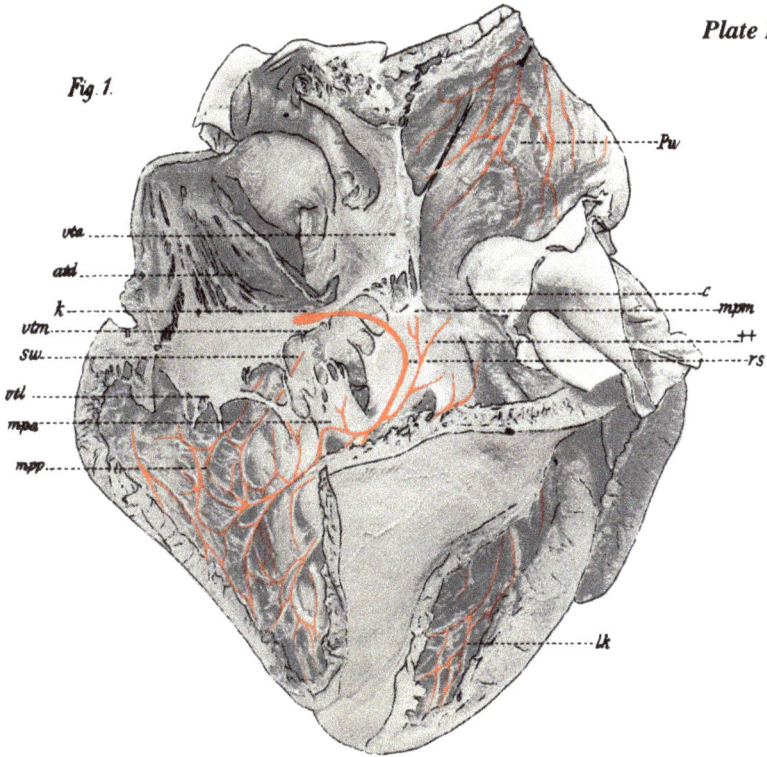

Fig. 2.

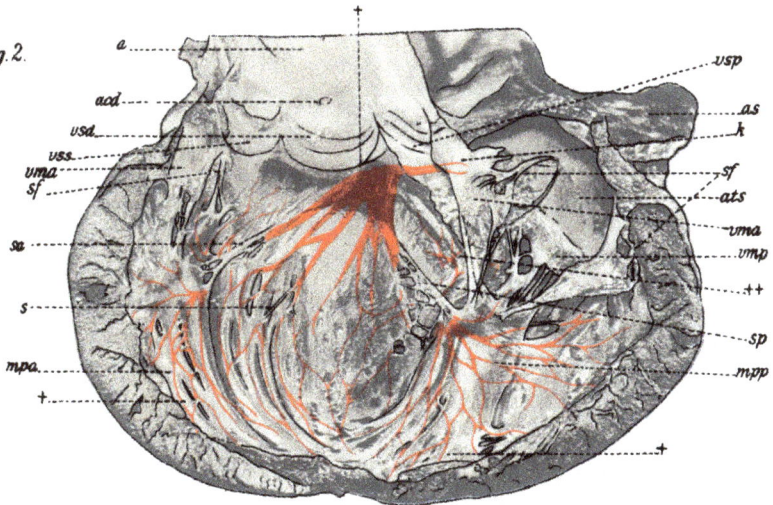

Plate III

Fig. 1.

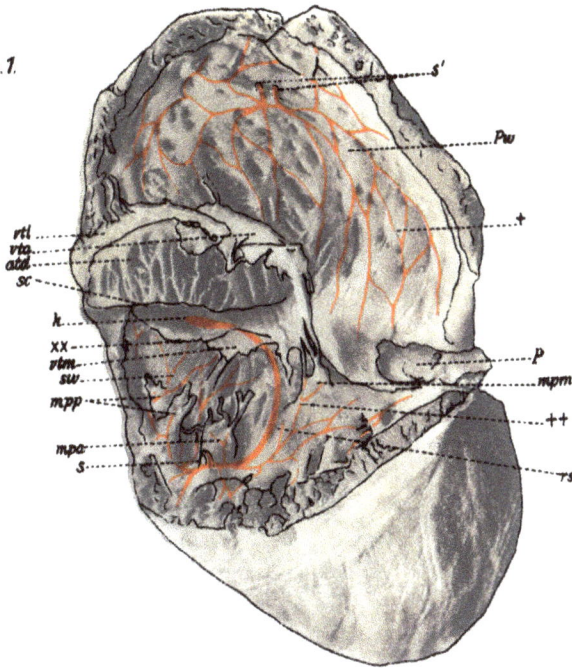

Fig 2.

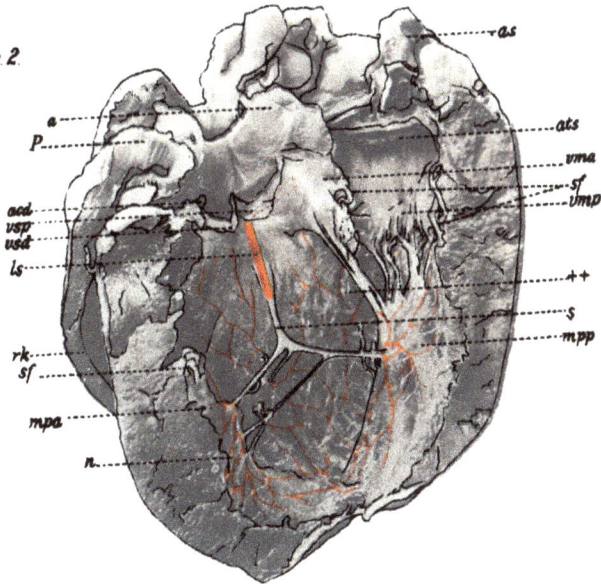

Fig.1.

Plate IV

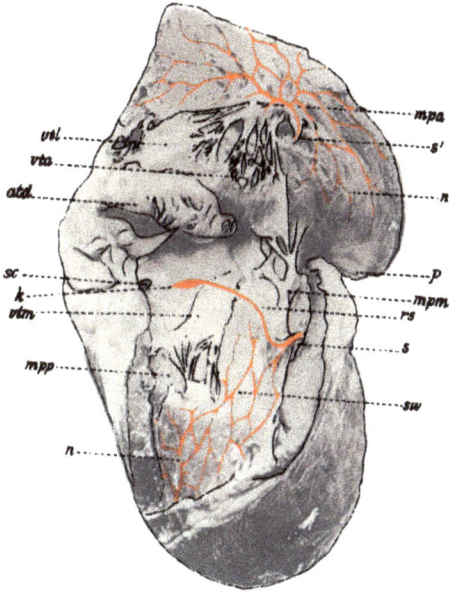

vtl
vta
atd

sc
k
vtm

mpp

n

mpa
s'
n

p
mpm
rs
s

sw

Fig.2.

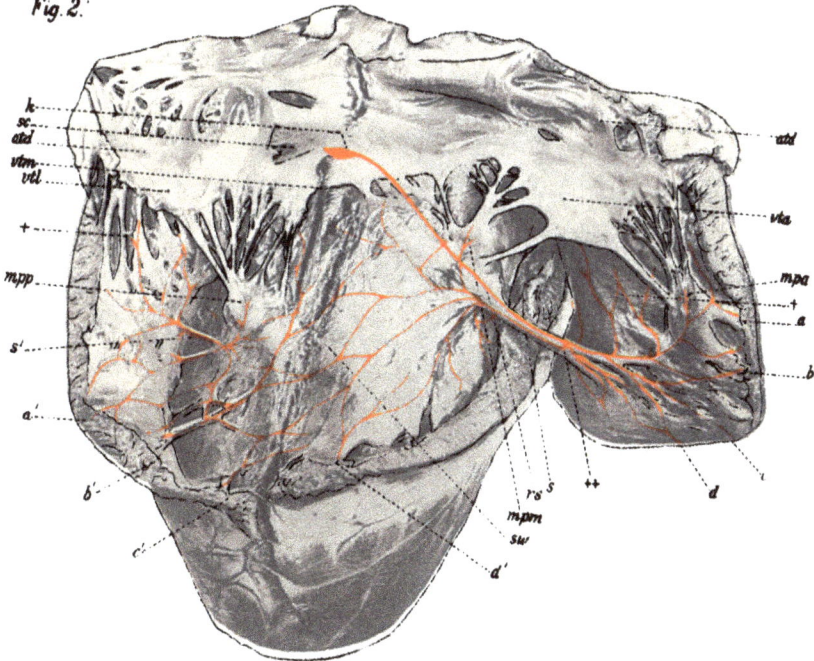

k
sc
atd
vtm
vtl

+

mpp

s'

a'

b'

c'

atd

vta

mpa
+
a

b

d

rs
s
++
mpm
sw
d'

Plate V

Fig 1.

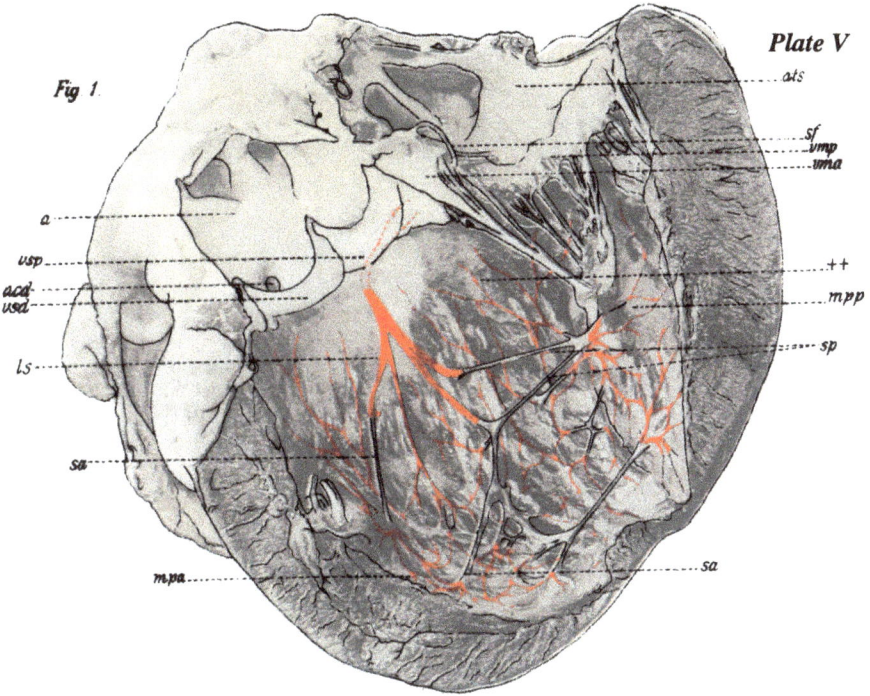

ats

sf
vmp
vma

a

vsp

acd
vsd

++

mpp

sp

ls

sa

sa

mpa

Fig. 2.

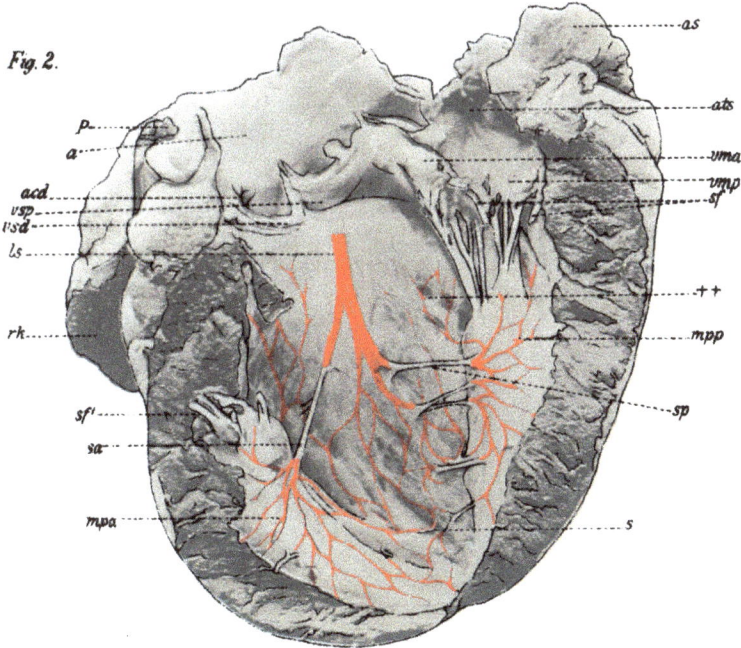

as

ats

p

a

vma

vmp

acd

sf

vsp

vsd

ls

++

rk

mpp

sf¹

sp

sa

mpa

s

References

(If the title of a paper is not given in a reference, it has been indicated in the text of this book.)

1. Krehl, *Deutsches Archiv für klinische Medizin*, Bd XLVI, S. 457.
2. E. Albrecht, Der Herzmuskel und seine Bedeutung für Physiologie, Pathologie und Klinik des Herzens (Berlin, 1903).
3. L. Aschoff, Zur Myokarditisfrage, in *Verhandlungen der Deutschen pathologischen Gesellschaft* (September 1904).
4. G. Paladino, Centribuzione all' anatomia, istologia e fisiologia del cuore, *Movimento med.-chirurg* (1876).
5. Bardeleben, *Jahresberichte für Anatomie und Physiologie* (1876), S. 251.
6. Gaskell, On the Innervation of the Heart, with Especial Reference to the Heart of the Tortoise, *Journal of Physiology* (1883), p. 43.
7. A. F. Stanley Kent, Researches on the Structure and Functions of the Mammalian Heart, *Journal of Physiology* (1893), Vol. XIV, p. 233.
8. Wilhelm His jun., *Arbeiten aus der med. Klinik zu Leipzig* (1893), S. 14–49.
9. R. Retzer, Über die muskulöse Verbindung zwischen Vorhof und Ventrikel des Säugetierherzens, *Archiv f. Anatomie u. Physiologie, Anatomische Abteilung* (1904), S. 1.
10. K. Braeunig, Über muskulöse Verbindung zwischen Vorkammer und Kammer bei verschiedenen Wirbeltierherzen, Inaugural-Dissertation (Berlin, 1904).

11. H. Schridde, Die Protoplasmafasern der menschlichen Epidermiszellen, *Archiv für mikroscopische Anatomie und Entwicklungsgeschichte* (1905), Bd. 67, S. 291.

12. A. v. Kölliker, Handbuch der Gewebslehre des Menschen, 6. Aufl., Bd. III, S. 612.

13. J. E. Purkinje, Mikroscopisch-neurologische Beobachtung, *Arch für Anatomie, Physiologie und wissenschaftliche Medizin* (Jahrg., 1845).

14. A. v. Kölliker, Handbuch der Gewebslehre (1852), S. 67.

15. T. v. Heßling, Histologische Mitteilungen, *Zeitschrift für weissenschaftliche Zoologie von C. T. Siebolt und A. Kölliker* (1854), V. Bd., S. 189.

16. C. B. Reichert, *Archiv für Anatomie, Physiologie und wissenschaftliche Medizin* (1885), S. 51.

17. R. Remak, *Archiv für Anatomie, Physiologie und wissenschaftliche Medizin* (1862), S. 230.

18. Ch. Aeby, Über die Bedeutung der Purkinjeschen Fäden, *Zeitschrift für rationale Medizin* (1863), Bd. XVII, 3. Reihe, S. 195.

19. C. J. Eberth, *Archiv für pathologische Anatomie und Physiologie und für klinische Medizin von Virchow* (1886), XXXVII. Bd., 3. Folge: VII. Bd., S. 100.

20. Obermeier, *Archiv für Anatomie, Physiologie und wissenschaftliche Medizin* (1867), S. 245 bis 255 und 358 bis 386.

21. M. Lehnert, *Archiv für mikroskopische Anatomie von Schultze* (1868), IV. Bd., S. 26.

22. A. Frisch, Zur Kenntnis der Purkinjeschen Fäden, *Sitzungsberichte d. Wiener Akademie, mathematisch-naturwissenschaftliche Klasse* (1869), LX. Bd., S. 341.

23. C. Gegenbauer, Notiz über das Vorkommen der Purkinjeschen Fäden, *Morphologisches Jahrbuch von Gegenbauer* (1877), III. Bd., S. 633.

24. R. Schmalz, *Archiv für wissenschaftliche u. praktische Tierheilkunde* (1886), XII. Bd., S. 161.

25. R. Minervini, *Anatomischer Anzeiger* (1899), Bd. XV, No. 1.

26. V. v. Ebner, *Sitzungsberichte der Wiener Akademie; mathematisch-naturwissenschaft-liche Klasse* (1900), CIX. Bd., Abt. III, S. 700.

27. H. Hoyer, *Anzeiger der Akademie der Wissenschaften in Krakau, mathematisch-naturwissenschaftliche Klasse* (1901), S. 205.

28. M. F. Marceau, Recherches sur l'histologie et le développement comparés des fibres de Purkinje et des fibres cardiaques, *Comptes Rendus de la Société de Biologie* (1901), S. 653.

29. H. K. Hofmann, *Zeitschrift für wissenschaftliche Zoologie* (1902), Bd. LXXI, Heft 3, S. 486.

30. G. Moriya, *Anatomischer Anzeiger* (1904), Bd. XXIV, S. 523.

31. T. W. Engelmann, *Die Deutsche Klinik* Bd. IV, S. 215.

32. G. Fano, *Arch. per le sc. med.* (1890), XIV.

33. H. E. Hering, Über die Erregungsleitung zwischen Vorkammer und Kammer des Säugetierherzens, *Archiv für die gesamte Physiologie* (1905), Bd. CVII, S. 106.

Name Index

Subject Index

Summary of the Results

Instructions Regarding the Method of Cutting the Atrioventricular Bundle in Animal Experiments

www.ingramcontent.com/pod-product-compliance
Lightning Source LLC
Chambersburg PA
CBHW050554190326

41458CB00007B/2033

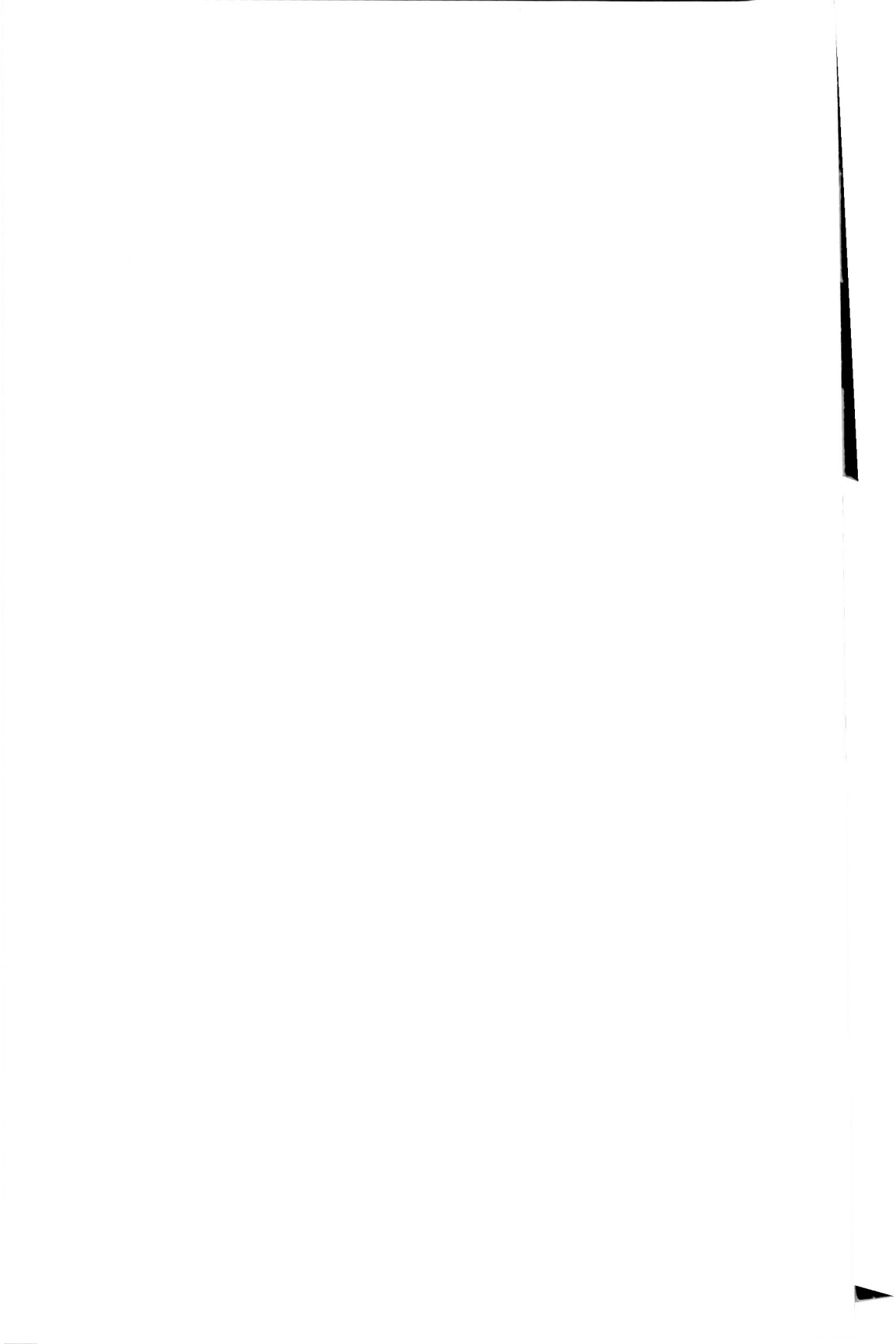